SLEEP SECRETS

th

DATE			

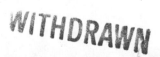

SLEEP SECRETS

for
Shift Workers & People with
Off-Beat Schedules

David Morgan

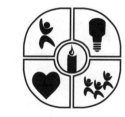

WHOLE PERSON ASSOCIATES
Duluth, Minnesota

Sleep Secrets for Shift Workers & People with Off-Beat Schedules

Printed in the United States of America
10 9 8 7 6 5 4 3

Editorial Director: Susan Gustafson
Graphic Design: Jeff Brownell
Manuscript Editor: Kathy DeArmond-Lundblad

Library of Congress Cataloging in Publication Data
Morgan, David R. (David Rees), 1930–
Sleep secrets for shift workers and people with off-beat schedules
   / by David Morgan.
   p.   cm.
   Includes bibliographical references.
   ISBN 1057025-118-5 (pbk. : acid-free paper)
   1. Sleep—Popular works. 2. Sleep disorders—Popular works.
   3. Shift systems—Health aspects.   I. Title.
RA786.M67 1996   96-9961
612.8'21—dc20   CIP

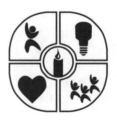

WHOLE PERSON ASSOCIATES
210 W Michigan
Duluth MN 55802-1908
800-247-6789

Table of contents

Foreword

After reading *Sleep Secrets for Shift Workers & People with Off-Beat Schedules,* I only wished it had been available two decades earlier when I was working as a young doctor. In the 1970s, a debilitating sleep debt was considered an essential right of passage for the apprenticing physician, providing, as it did, an opportunity to experience most aspects of medical practice "around the clock." Having received no instruction during my medical training on the importance of sleep—in either health or disease—and not being particularly wise, I and my colleagues assumed that dozing whilst assisting at surgery or falling asleep whilst conversing or eating was the mark of being a good doctor in demand rather than a sign of pathological and perilous sleep deprivation.

Although the guardians of public safety now realize that sleep loss is dangerous and have required medical training programs to limit the hours of extra duty for doctors, unfamiliarity about sleep, generally, and how to manage shift work, particularly, remains widespread both amongst the public and the medical profession. In our schools, education about sleep is usually limited to descriptions of the stages of sleep and dreaming with practical information about preventing protracted sleep loss and its potentially deadly consequences amongst our youngest drivers being rarely offered.

Unfortunately, the education of health professionals is not much better: My generation of doctors rarely received any instruction about sleep. In the 1980s, specific sleep disorders were being identified and treatments defined, but it wasn't until 1989 that the first comprehensive textbook on sleep disorders for health professionals was published. Despite the recent yet rapid growth in knowledge about sleep and its disorders, medical schools have been slow to include this information in their curricula. It has been estimated that most medical schools give less than two hours of instruction on sleep to their students, and consequently, the distressed poor sleeper may have to search far and wide to obtain appropriate assistance.

Given the widespread prevalence of shift work and its known effects on sleep and health, there is a need for an easily read, factual, and practical guide to help shift workers adapt to the demands of this special type of work. A number of research studies have demonstrated that simply providing workers who must sleep at unusual times with information about good sleep hygiene significantly improves their sleep and their adaptation to and enjoyment from life. For some shift workers this will be sufficient; others will require more assistance and information about their difficulties.

Anyone interested in the process of sleep and its associated disorders will learn from reading this well written, self-help book. As there is much to be gleaned from its pages, it should be required reading for both the novice and seasoned shift worker. The author carefully directs the reader through a practical, straightforward, step-by-step approach to identifying the issues associated with shift work and then reviews potential solutions for these problems. Although I could not benefit from this book during my short career as a shift worker I highly recommend it to others and shall ask all my patients who must cope with the special demands of shift work to read it.

Dr. Jonathan A. E. Fleming, M.B., F.R.C.P.(C)
Co-Director, Sleep Disorders Program
Vancouver Hospital and Health Sciences Centre, UBC Site
Vancouver
Canada

STEP 1

RECOGNIZE THE PROBLEM:

IT CAN BE LETHAL

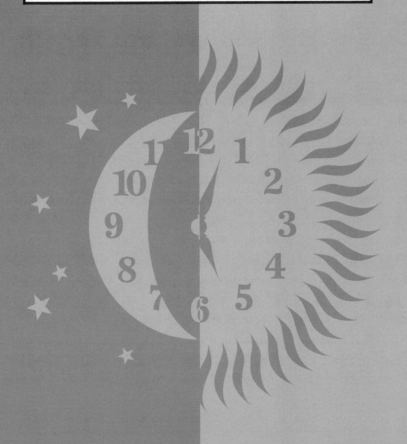

1

When you work shifts, getting sleep is a survival skill —your life is at stake!

I looked at the grim blackened wreckage strewn over one hundred feet of desert rock and sand alongside Interstate 40 in eastern California. I found it hard to imagine that it had once been an eighteen-wheeler truck. I could see no trace of what it had been carrying. It may have been empty, or maybe its freight had burned up. There was no sign of a cab in the black, mangled metal. One thing was clear: the truck had been driven off the highway on to the shoulder at cruising speed. There was no sign of any attempt to slow down; there were no skid marks. The driver may have had a heart attack and lost control of his rig that way. But most likely he fell asleep.

His last moments can be imagined: the sudden, violent jolting as the tractor's front wheels crossed the shoulder shocked the driver awake immediately, but his attempt to regain control came about two seconds too late, just as the front wheels dug into the soft ground. That slowed the tractor, while the trailer behind, pushing ahead at sixty miles per hour, jackknifed over the cab, crushed the driver instantly, and burst the fuel tank. Flames then engulfed the wreckage. All this in about twenty seconds from the time the driver nodded off.

It made me sad to think that this driver, a shift worker, probably died for the lack of something as simple as a few hours sleep. Like air to breathe and water to drink, sleep is a need that can be satisfied without spending a cent. But unlike your body's demands for air and water, the demand for sleep can be put off, just as you might put off paying back a loan.

Sleep is like an easygoing but moody banker. At first he lets you borrow all the time that you want, allowing your sleep debt to grow bigger. Then suddenly he demands payment in sleep, often at a very inconvenient or even dangerous time. And he will take that sleep payment even at the cost of your life. This "banker" can be very dangerous—especially for shift workers.

Your shift work brings irregular sleep times, daytime noise, job pressures, and family pressures, so learning how to get enough sleep—how to deal with your "banker"—is vital for your health and happiness. But more than that, it is a survival skill.

Tackling a major, but neglected, problem

Everyone has heard of jet lag; who has heard of "shift lag"? Jet lag, a sleep problem that affects a relatively small number of air travelers for a very short time, gets a lot of attention. But the sleep problems of shift workers, which affect a very large population year after year, have been strangely neglected.

One of every four men and one of every six women in the United States is a shift worker; approximately 25 million Americans work shifts. According to one study, half of them have sleep problems.

People most likely to be working shifts, according to a U.S. Bureau of Labor survey, are as follows:

- Protective services (firefighters, police, security): 61 percent

- Food services (cooks, waiters, waitresses): 43 percent

- Health services: (nurses, paramedics, doctors): 36 percent

- Factory workers, retail sales clerks, labor: 25 percent

But these statistics give just a glimpse of the huge numbers of different types of shift workers, working a great variety of shift systems, all the way from regular clockwork shift systems to every variety of irregular working hours that you can imagine.

As a shift worker, you might be:

- An actor, performing on stage or in a TV studio or night club

- An air traffic controller, watching radar blips as you guide aircraft safely through the dark

- A radio or TV broadcaster, keeping your station on the air while you entertain a night owl audience

- A short order cook, feeding other shift workers in an all-night restaurant

- A cabbie, waiting for a late night call and glad to hear a fellow shift worker give you the news and weather on your radio

- A cleaner, sweeping and scrubbing your way through giant office buildings while the office staff sleep far away

- A college student, working evenings or nights while trying to keep up on studies and still get enough sleep

- A construction worker, always under pressure to get the job done, day or night.

- A convenience store clerk, glad to see a customer late at night but also a little nervous about holdups

- A driller on a diamond drill or oil rig, handling heavy equipment in all weather, night or day, on lonely jobs

- A flight attendant, trying to be bright, cheerful, courteous, and helpful with often tired and cranky passengers

- A highway worker, struggling to keep roads open through an all-night snowfall

- A journalist, up late or early to get a story or meet a deadline

- A miner, drilling and blasting underground, where night always lasts twenty-four hours

- A police officer, driving a late, routine patrol, which may suddenly stop being routine

■ A waitress and single mom, worrying throughout the night about her kids asleep at home

Shift work is almost as old as the human race. Guards and night watchmen go as far back as history itself; ships have operated on a watch system for many hundreds of years; for centuries mines have also operated around the clock, since day is as dark as night underground. But within the last one hundred years, shift work has increased enormously. Electric light made night work possible on a large scale. Modern industry must go nonstop to be more profitable. Many industries, such as steel production, cannot operate with interruptions.

Shift work is a fact of life today. Our society cannot function without it. It is also a fact of life that shift work can have bad effects on the shift worker's health. "Compared with permanent day workers, rotating shift workers have a higher incidence of sleep disorders and gastrointestinal complaints, including ulcers," says sleep researcher M. C. Moore-Ede. Other effects of long-term shift work appear in a Swedish study, which indicates that the risk of coronary artery disease doubles after five years of rotating shift work and triples after ten years.

The difficulties and stresses of shift work all come from a simple and obvious fact: it is not natural to work at night and sleep during the day. When you oppose nature in this way, you often are drowsy or half asleep on the job and half awake when you want to rest. For shift workers, therefore, sleep is a central problem.

In this chapter you will see some of the dangers of being asleep at the wheel and asleep on the job. The following chapters will show you how your sleep problems can be solved and how you can protect your health and maybe even your life as a shift worker by taking advantage of recent sleep research discoveries.

Shift work dangers: asleep at the wheel

The Tuba City School bus with thirty children (ages five to twenty-one) on board had stopped near Tuba City, about twenty-five miles east of the Grand Canyon, Arizona, at 3:15 P.M. on April 29, 1985.

A tractor-semitrailer hit the bus from behind, killing two children and seriously injuring four. Only four children escaped injury. The drivers of the bus and of the truck had minor injuries. The National Transportation Safety Board (NTSB) investigation showed that the accident was due to the truck driver's lack of sleep. The truck driver was found to have kept one logbook for his company and one for himself. Entries in these logs did not match. The night before the accident the driver had slept from 10:00 P.M. to 3:30 A.M. on the floor of a motel room that he shared with other truck drivers. The NTSB found that the driver worked long hours and had an irregular duty pattern. The immediate causes of his accident were easily seen; in the background, less easily seen were the work pressures that most truckers endure.

Accidents of this type are not rare. Studies show that as many as 6,500 highway deaths in the U.S. in one year may be due to a driver falling asleep. In another study, 15 percent of the shift workers questioned reported falling asleep driving at least once every three months. The problem is also worldwide. The Leicestershire police in Britain see sleepiness as the cause of 20 percent of all highway accidents. British authorities attribute 5 percent of truck accidents to sleepy drivers. In Japan, one study placed the rate at 9 percent. Accidents of this type are also particularly deadly, since the driver makes no attempt to slow down or avoid trees, cliffs, or other vehicles. These accidents account for 45 percent of all traffic deaths, according to the Japanese study. A study of all car accidents over a six-year period in Israel supported this finding. It showed that sleep-related highway accidents were three times more likely to result in death or serious injury compared to other accidents.

Irregular hours and fierce competition put great pressure on truck drivers to keep working when they need rest, but even workers on regular shifts fall asleep in spite of great risks. A pilot fell asleep during a landing while his aircraft was only two hundred feet above the ground; the copilot wakened him just in time to land safely. More surprising than this was the case of the Boeing 707 airliner, westbound to Los Angeles, that continued past the city for one hundred miles over the Pacific on autopilot with all three pilots fast asleep. Air traffic controllers were finally successful in triggering cockpit alarms and waking the crew while the plane still had enough fuel to return.

Not so lucky were the crews of two Burlington Northern freight trains that collided head-on sixty miles northeast of Denver at 3:58 A.M. on April 13, 1984. Five crew members died and two were injured in this accident, which destroyed seven locomotives and twenty-six freight cars and did $3.9 million damage. The National Transportation Safety Board found that the probable cause was that the engineer and other head-end crew members of one of the trains fell asleep. Voluntary lack of sleep, consumption of alcohol, and an irregular shift system with changing work/rest cycles were all important causes of this disaster.

Irregular shifts, however, were not the cause of the grounding of the Japanese tankship *Matsukaze* in the Strait of Juan de Fuca, eighty miles northwest of Seattle. The second mate was on fixed, regular daily shifts from midnight to 4:00 A.M. and from noon to 4:00 P.M. He had regular living conditions and meals, a familiar cabin to sleep in, and the clockwork routines of a ship at sea to support him. Nevertheless, on April 28, 1988, while on duty alone on the bridge, he fell asleep at about 2:30 A.M. The ship went aground at 3:15 A.M. This accident shows that even strictly disciplined shift workers working routine shifts are at risk.

It is vital for you as a shift worker to learn the survival skills of getting the sleep you need. You never know when that sleep "banker" will call in his sleep loan. He is ruthless. He doesn't care about the fate of a sleepy ship's officer who runs the ship aground, or a shift worker driving home who dozes off while the traffic lights are red, or even a truck driver who is cruising along at sixty miles per hour who just happens to nod off for a few seconds.

Shift work dangers: asleep on the job

Falling asleep while working at the controls of any moving vehicle, whether on land, at sea, or in the air, usually leads to disaster. Other shift work jobs may be less deadly. Sleeping or sleepy shift workers are more likely to be less productive than destructive.

But industrial accidents in which the strains of shift work are a factor can be very serious, too. In the nuclear power industry, for instance, sleepy workers have contributed to disasters far greater than any transportation accident. Lack of sleep is suspected in night shift errors leading to the Three Mile Island (1979) and the Chernobyl (1986) nuclear power plant disasters; it also played a part in serious reactor incidents at Oak Harbor, Ohio (1985), and Rancho Seco near Sacramento (1985). In August 1988 the U.S. Nuclear Regulatory Commission shut down the Peach Bottom Nuclear Reactor in Pennsylvania after operators were found sleeping on duty. The company was fined $1.25 million for negligence. Charles Czeisler, head of the Center for Design of Industrial Schedules in Boston, found that of the nuclear power plant operators questioned, half reported falling asleep on the job.

Similarly, "operator fatigue" was cited as a major factor in a near catastrophic launch of the space shuttle *Columbia* on January 6, 1986. On that occasion, console operators mistakenly drained nine tons of vital liquid oxygen fuel from the shuttle's external tanks within five minutes of lift-off. Luckily, the lift-off was canceled in the last thirty-one seconds due to an engine malfunction. Just three weeks later, faulty decisions made by key managers, short on sleep, contributed to the *Challenger* shuttle disaster, according to a presidential commission.

It seems, then, that lack of sleep can cause inefficiency, problems, and disasters, even in high-tech nuclear power and space sectors where every resource is made available. It is, therefore, not surprising that the efficiency of millions of shift workers in less glamorous jobs is affected.

A 1988 article in the *Wall Street Journal* estimated that the financial cost of shift work in reduced alertness, productivity, and safety amounted to about $70 billion a year. Many detailed studies provide support for such estimates. A study of one group of shift workers indicated that half of them fall asleep on the job at least once a week. In Sweden, researchers had the workers at a paper mill wear electrical brain wave recorders (electroencephalograph, or EEG) over a forty-eight-hour period. The study showed that one-fifth of them fell asleep between 2 A.M. and 4 A.M. for an average of about forty-five minutes while sitting in chairs. The workers said that they were "dozing off," but the EEG readings showed that 32 percent of their "dozing" was deep sleep.

Shift workers are often half awake or asleep on the job mainly because they are often half asleep or wide awake in bed. The next section looks at the sleep wreckers waiting for the shift workers as they head for bed after a long graveyard shift.

A shift work problem: wide awake in bed

If you work on a night shift from midnight to 8 A.M., you will go to bed just as daylight is getting up towards full strength. Between you and the rest that you need so badly can stand a big lineup of sleep wreckers, many of them unknown to people who don't work shifts.

The first sleep wrecker to visit you may be the Graveyard Hangover. Night shifts can be quiet and dull, but many are not. If you have spent the shift fighting a fire, driving a truck through heavy traffic, attending to nervous passengers on a long flight, or working as a nurse in a busy hospital emergency room, you probably need a chance to unwind. People who work nine-to-five have six hours to unwind before bedtime. Shift workers often have to schedule their day sleep without allowing time to "switch off the job." If you didn't find a chance to relax, talk it out, and laugh it off, the tensions of a long, hard night shift can be a very effective daytime sleep wrecker.

The next sleep wrecker waiting for you may be Strange Surroundings. Your room and the bed that you are trying to sleep in may be strange ones. If you are a trucker, a pilot, a flight attendant, or a member of a train crew, you will often sleep far from home, in a bed and a room that you have never seen before. You may have no time to move from a hot, noisy room with a lumpy bed to one that is more comfortable, or the room you're in may be the best that is available. If you work shifts as a construction worker, a driller, a miner, a sailor, or a member of the armed forces, you may also sleep far from home and find that you have little choice in the beds and bedrooms offered to you.

Even if you escape these first two sleep wreckers, you will almost certainly get a visit from Daytime Noise. It will bring you roaring traffic outside, a road crew with a growling compressor and clattering drills down the street, whining vacuum cleaners and babbling TV sitcoms in the surrounding rooms or apartments, and a phone ready to ring just two feet from your head. Our civilization depends on shift workers, but it doesn't show them much mercy when they are trying to sleep during the day.

Then there is a sturdy gang called the Ever Ready sleep wreckers, ever ready to show up and wreck your sleep whatever shift you are on. Those false friends alcohol and sleeping pills belong to this gang. They may bring unconsciousness, but that is a very different thing from healthy sleep. Also in this gang are worry, regret, and guilt—always ready to wreck your sleep if you let them.

But the strongest and in some ways the strangest of these sleep wreckers is one that you carry with you wherever you go. Its name is Body Clock. A loudly ticking old-fashioned alarm clock can keep you awake; so can your body's own quiet internal clock. If you understand this internal clock and treat it with respect, it will serve you well; ignore it or neglect it, and you may be wide awake when you want to sleep and nodding off just when you are trying to stay awake. Your body clock regulates most of your body's housekeeping arrangements, such as digestion, temperature, the ebb and flow of your energy, and, last but not least, your sleep cycles. When you go on night shift your body clock at first will have everything backwards. It will turn on your energy in the morning when you want to sleep and it will turn your energy down to a low point at about 4 A.M., when your job may well demand your full alertness. Of all the sleep wreckers, this one is the most important to understand and control.

This book will show you how to deal with all of these sleep wreckers so that you sleep better, survive shift work, and maybe even enjoy it.

STEP 2

ANALYZE THE PROBLEM: IS IT ONE FOR YOUR DOCTOR?

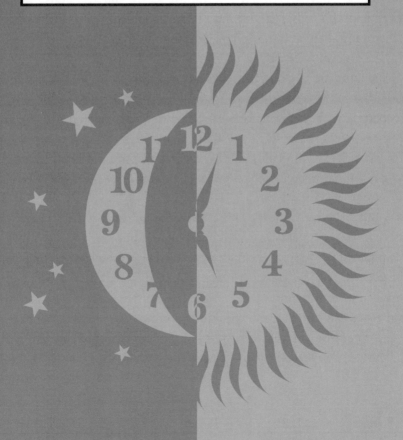

2

How to identify
your sleep problem
when you work shifts

You lie down on a comfortable bed, put your head on a soft pillow, and close your eyes. In a few minutes, you have a sensation of falling, and you begin drifting off into a sound sleep. That's how sleep should come to us, but quite often the experience is different, especially for shift workers.

Why is sleep, something so natural and so important to your health, sometimes so difficult to get? Part of the answer is that falling asleep is different from almost anything else that you do. If you are hungry, you find food and eat it; if you are thirsty, you get something to drink; if you are cold, you light a fire or put on a coat. In short, when you want to satisfy a basic need, you do something about it. You take action.

But sleep is different. Sleep means switching off action. In fact, the solution to most sleep problems consists of mainly removing the things that prevent sleep. Your body knows how to sleep. Once you remove the obstacles, your body will take over. Most of this book presents ways to help you get rid of the sleep wreckers in your life, starting with the easy ones and then moving on to the tougher cases.

Before you start, however, it is very important to find out if all or part of your sleep problem calls for your doctor's help. This is not a medical textbook, but it can help you decide if you need medical help.

Then you will meet the team who designed your sleep system. If the world today seems like a wild and dangerous place, you will be glad to learn that your cave-dwelling ancestors spent a lot of time perfecting a sleep system designed specially for a dangerous world. They passed on a top-of-the-line system to you.

Finally, this chapter looks at the "Olympic champions" of the sleep world: people whose sleep is of such high quality that they need far less than eight hours. The skills of these "athletes" may be pointing to a future of shorter, higher quality sleep for the rest of us.

Is your sleep problem one for your doctor?

Many medical sleep problems must be treated by a doctor or a sleep specialist. In this section you'll find the symptoms of some of the more common medical sleep problems. If you have any of these symptoms, you should see your doctor.

The list below certainly does not cover the symptoms of every possible sleep problem that should be treated by your doctor, so the rule is, if in doubt, see your doctor.

Sleep apnea

1. You are often exhausted, although you have been "asleep" for eight hours.

2. You are a heavy snorer.

3. You are probably overweight.

4. Your snoring is often interrupted and your breathing stops. Then after 30–120 seconds, with a big gasp, your breathing and your snoring begin again.

5. You keep having these interruptions in your breathing during the night, sometimes as often as every few minutes.

6. You may not even realize that these repeated, exhausting interruptions to your sleep are happening.

If these symptoms describe your sleep problem, you may have sleep apnea. Untreated, this malady, which is already ruining your sleep, can be fatal. So if you suspect that you may have it, you must see your doctor. (Note: If you sleep alone and have symptoms 1, 2, and 3, try leaving a tape recorder recording while you sleep. If the playback sounds like symptom 4, take the tape to your doctor.)

Narcolepsy

1. You are sleepy most of the time and not only find it easy to fall asleep but sometimes do so suddenly while you are talking, eating, or even driving.

2. When you are excited by laughter, anger, fear, or sadness, you may suddenly fall fast asleep without being able to prevent it.

3. When you are excited by laughter, anger, fear, or sadness, you may suddenly lose the strength of your muscles and stagger, fall over, or drop things. You are wide awake when this happens, but you can do nothing to prevent it. (This sudden temporary paralysis is called cataplexy.)

4. When you wake up or while you are going to sleep, you are unable to move for seconds or even minutes. This short-lasting paralysis can be very alarming.

5. You have strong and very real dreams while you are awake, or you have very powerful, bad dreams just as you are dropping off to sleep.

If you have any of these symptoms you may have narcolepsy, and you should see your doctor. Narcolepsy is not always easy to detect. New symptoms may appear as time passes, and since you may suddenly fall asleep while walking across the street or driving a car, narcolepsy can be dangerous.

Involuntary muscle contractions

1. You are often exhausted, although you have been "asleep" for eight hours.

2. While you sleep, you are kicking every few minutes. You may not be aware of this, but it is disturbing your sleep and leaving you exhausted. If this describes your case, you may be a kicker. If so, see your doctor.

(Note: If you sleep alone and have symptom 1, try leaving a tape recorder going while you sleep. If the playback sounds like symptom 2, take the tape to your doctor)

Depression

1. Your life always seems grey and drab, even when the sun is shining. The past seems desolate, the present is dull, and the future looks hopeless.

2. Nothing really interests you, and it is hard to concentrate on anything.

3. You have no appetite for food or sex; you have little energy.

4. You are often unable to sleep, and when you do it is a shallow sleep. You never seem to have a deep, refreshing sleep.

5. You have been like this for several weeks or even months.

If this describes your symptoms, you may be suffering from depression. You should see your doctor.

Night shift paralysis

1. You are a nurse, air traffic controller, naval officer, or printer or have some other job where your work involves heavy responsibilities and exact attention to details.

2. Your shift system is burdensome, often requires you to work two or more night shifts in a row, and sometimes involves working a morning and a night shift on the same day.

3. When you are not working shifts, you tend to come to life towards the end of the day and be an "evening person." You also tend to have more difficulty than most people at getting used to new sleep times.

4. Sometimes when you are on night shift (especially around 5:00 A.M.) you find that although you are wide awake, you are paralyzed and unable to move for a few seconds, or even as long as a few minutes. This may have happened to you only once, or it may have happened on several shifts.

If this describes your symptoms, you may have experienced night shift paralysis. You should see your doctor.

Other problems that require medical attention

You should see your doctor if you have any sleep problems and also:

1. You have heart problems, high blood pressure, asthma, arthritis, diabetes, or other illness or chronic condition.

2. You are recovering from an injury or operation.

3. You have constant or repeated pain.

4. You are taking a medication prescribed by your doctor.

5. Substance abuse (drugs, smoking, or alcohol) has an important place in your life.

Your smart sleep system: it's designed for a wild world

Imagine that you are living on the plains of East Africa long ago. Tall grass and small stands of flat-topped thorn trees cover the mostly flat country. In the hazy distance rises a giant snow-capped volcano. Game is plentiful: gazelle, antelope, zebra roam, along with giraffe, elephants, lions, and packs of wild dogs. You live with about fifty other people in a small village among some big boulders. Through the evening you have been sitting in a group around an open fire, going over the events of the day. Now you are tired and you want to go to sleep. It is probably safe to sleep for a while, but you know that your sleep may be disturbed by prowling animals, so from time to time you will wake up and see what is happening. If all is well, you will go back to sleep.

Human beings much like us lived like this for about three million years, maybe more. If you think of the story of the human race as being twenty-four hours long, we lived like this in little tribes until three minutes ago. Reading, writing, the invention of the wheel, ancient Babylon, Columbus, and jet planes; all happened in the last three minutes.

This means that our sleep habits were mostly formed under prehistoric conditions during hundreds of thousands of years. Back then, to sink into a deep sleep for several hours was probably dangerous. Anyone who slept like that probably didn't survive. The wild dogs or the lions got them.

Most animals in the wild are cautious sleepers, waking frequently to make sure all is well. Chimpanzees in the wild typically sleep a bit more than nine and a half hours between dusk and dawn, but wake frequently for as long as an hour, with a total awake time of about an hour and a half. In a tribe of sleeping chimpanzees , one or two are awake to sound an alarm if need be.

Our background probably accounts for the cautious way we sleep now. When you fall asleep, you plunge toward the deep sleep you need to nourish and restore your brain. It will usually take you about half an hour to get down to this deep sleep, and you will remain in it for about forty-five minutes. In this sleep you are difficult to wake and tend to sleep through disturbances that would wake you in shallower sleep.

Then it is almost as if it is time to surface to see if all is well. So you rapidly leave this deep sleep and come almost to the surface of wakefulness. But usually, instead of waking up, you begin to dream. Anyone watching your face during this stage of light sleep will see your eyeballs move rapidly this way and that beneath the closed lids. For that reason this sleep stage is called "rapid eye movement," or REM, sleep.

Then after about ten minutes of REM sleep, you plunge back down again to deep sleep. From one plunge to the next takes about ninety minutes. You will take about five of these ninety-minute sleep plunges during a normal eight-hour sleep. So your ninety-minute cycle gives you a mix of all of the types of sleep that you need, and then brings you back up to a shallow sleep where you are easily woken. If all is well, you will then plunge back down for some more deep sleep. Even if you only manage to get ninety minutes sleep before, for instance, you have to get up, jump on a fire truck, and put out a fire, you will have had a "balanced diet" of sleep.

Knowing about two aspects of these ninety-minute sleep cycles can help you with your sleep problems today. First, these ninety-minute sleep cycles are a very deeply planted and successful design for sleep. Each cycle contains deep sleep and REM sleep, both of which are essential for healthy rest. Anything that upsets these cycles causes you sleep troubles. Some people who suffer from depression are unable to get to the deep sleep in their sleep cycle. Lack of this deep sleep makes them even more depressed. Medical assistance may be needed to break this cycle. Many drugs interfere with these cycles. Alcohol, for instance, suppresses REM sleep. When alcoholics try to quit drinking, the suppressed REM sleep bounces back with a vengeance. This REM rebound, as it is called, brings them such horrible dreams and even waking fantasies that they want to go back to alcohol to escape from them. But you can suffer from REM rebound without being an alcoholic. Some sleeping pills suppress REM sleep, and long-term users who quit can also suffer from the wild dreams of REM rebound. So protecting your natural sleep cycles is important.

Second, these cycles bring you repeated zones of light sleep, when you surface to see if all is well. This light sleep is where the roaring and snarling of your sleep wreckers may give you bad dreams or wake you up. (Our civilized life has threats and anxieties that easily match lions and packs of wild dogs.)

Banishing these enemies of good sleep is a survival skill. It is dealt with in a later chapter, called 'How to eliminate some of the worst enemies of sleep."

Short but higher-quality sleep: a design for the future?

Eight hours sleep in twenty-four is what most people need, but a seventy-year-old English nurse sleeps just one hour a night. She has slept like this all her life. How does she do it? Napoleon slept only four or five hours a night while he was conquering Europe. Thomas Edison, inventor of the electric light bulb, slept only four hours a night. The Russian leader Boris Yeltsin runs his troubled country on only three and a half hours of sleep each night.

Legends tend to grow around famous men so there is much we don't know about how Napoleon and Edison slept; they never had their sleep habits studied in a sleep laboratory. But the English nurse did. A researcher found, during a five-night study at the University of Technology in Loughborough, England, that she averaged sixty-seven minutes of sleep per night, took no naps, and showed no sign of fatigue during the day.

People who need only one hour of sleep per night are very uncommon, but three-to-four-hours-per-night sleepers are less rare. A University of Western Australia study described a fifty-four-year-old businessman and a thirty-four-year old draftsman who each slept only three hours per night.

How are these short sleepers able to do without the eight hours that most of us need? Part of the answer comes from a study of their brain waves while they sleep. The electroencephalograph (EEG), an instrument that displays and records the brain's electrical activity, is standard equipment in sleep laboratories. Since each stage of sleep has its own EEG pattern, or signature, it is possible to follow the sleeper's progress through the light, deep, and REM sleep of each ninety-minute sleep cycle.

Very short sleepers spend little time in the stages of light sleep. The EEG shows that they rapidly plunge down to deep sleep, spend most of their time there, and then climb rapidly up to REM sleep. It seems, then, that these naturally short sleepers are able to get the essential deep sleep and REM sleep they need in a short time; they are very efficient sleepers.

What is minimum sleep for normal people? The military is interested in knowing how long people can work continuously in emergency conditions. Tests showed that after three days of continuous work without sleep, members of a British parachute regiment were militarily ineffective. However, if these troops were

allowed even a small amount of sleep there was a huge improvement. With just ninety minutes of daily sleep, 50 percent of the
group was able to do nine days of continuous work. If daily sleep was
increased to three hours, 91 percent of the group was able to keep
working.

Is it possible to reduce your need for sleep and sleep more
efficiently? Can you cut down your sleep and still be rested and
refreshed? Yes, maybe you can, answers a University of San Diego
study. In this study, four couples in good physical and mental health,
all with jobs, wanted to reduce the time spent sleeping. They began
by cutting back thirty minutes every two weeks, until they were
sleeping six and a half hours a night. Then they cut back from six and
a half to five and a half hours by sleeping thirty minutes less every
three weeks. They progressed in this way, comfortably and always
able to work well. Results:

- None of the group could function with less than four and a
  half hours of sleep per night.

- For most of the group, six and a half hours of sleep is the
  bottom line.

- Six years after the study, four members of the group were
  sleeping an average of one and a half hours less per night.

Similar results have come from other researchers. So it does
seem to be possible to learn to sleep less. The eight-hour sleepers
seem to have trimmed off one and a half hours of what sleep
researcher James Horne calls "optional" sleep and are left with six
and a half hours of essential, or "core" sleep.

Perhaps these experiments are giving us a glimpse of the future—
a future where people have fewer anxieties, tensions, and frustra-
tions and live a higher quality life. Shorter but higher-quality sleep
may then offer more time to enjoy such a life.

STEP 3

FIX THE EASY THINGS FIRST

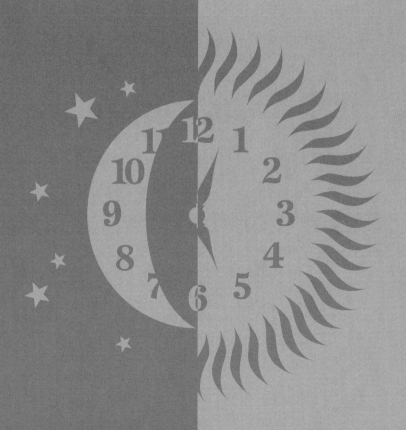

3

Changing your bedroom into a sleeproom

Bedrooms often become offices, sewing rooms, TV-watching rooms, reading rooms, and even junk rooms. Many bedrooms are too hot or too cold, stuffy, and never really quiet. Or they may be ugly, bare rooms if their owners don't see the point of being asleep in a beautiful room.

Take a fresh look at your bedroom. What disturbing, sleep-destroying objects do you tolerate in this important room in which you spend one third of your life? Is there a television set in there? Are there study books, news magazines, or newspapers on your bedside table? Do you sleep with a telephone a few feet from your head? Is a work desk or a sewing table part of the furniture? All of these items link your bedroom to special activities and make it that much less a sleeproom.

So it may be time to make some changes. This section will show you how to transform your bedroom into a sleeproom, simply and at little cost.

Create a comfortable bed

Beds come in great variety. Eskimos used to cut a raised shelf in the hard snow in their igloo, cover it with a caribou skin, and sleep comfortably on a block of ice. Russian peasants built the family bed over the stove in their cottages. King Louis XIV of France had 413 beds in his many palaces, including his great bed at the Palace of Versailles near Paris. This bed had crimson velvet curtains on which the "Triumph of Venus" was so richly embroidered in gold that little of the velvet showed. However, that was three hundred years ago, so Louis did not have flush toilets, central heating, or air conditioning. Also, fleas were looked as an acceptable nuisance in his palace. So as far as bodily comfort is concerned, anyone today can match the sleeproom of France's most extravagant king. You do not need 413 beds to sleep in; just one good one will do.

What makes a good bed? To allow a good night's sleep, your bed should be:

1. Big enough. Your bed should be big enough so that when you roll over (and people move from eight to thirty times during a night of sleep), you do not roll out of bed or disturb your partner. A sixty-inch-wide bed (queen size) is quite wide enough for two peaceful sleepers. If your partner or you are a restless sleeper, a seventy-six-inch wide bed (king size) may solve the problem. If not, separate beds may be the best solution.

2. Comfortable. Making a bed comfortable today is probably the easiest part of getting a good night's sleep. A fiercely competitive market waits out there, eager to supply you with a comfortable bed. Its comfort may come from a spring mattress, air mattress, cotton-stuffed futon, rubber sponge, plastic sponge, or the gentle waves of a water bed. Today, you do not have to tolerate an uncomfortable bed. Comfort is an essential that is easily achieved.

3. Warm. Using your muscles keeps you warm. When you sleep, the 639 muscles in your body stop moving. Only your heart and lung muscles keep working, and even these faithful servants take it easy during sleep. Since you are producing less heat, you need extra warmth from bedclothes. Your bedclothes probably get only a tiny part of the attention that the clothes in your closet get. This can be a mistake. You

spend a third of your life in bed, and the right bedclothes are important for good sleep. You can get some sleep in a bed that is too warm or too cold, but you don't sleep well and usually wake up sweating or shivering. The point is this: take some trouble to get the warmth of your bed just right. You will fall asleep more easily and sleep more soundly if you do. Again, a market stands ready to supply you with every conceivable way of keeping your bed warm (unless you insist on a caribou skin mattress or red velvet bed curtains richly embroidered with gold, and even those probably can be found!).

4. Dry. This is not as obvious as it may sound. We humans are surprisingly damp creatures. In a day you perspire about a quart of sweat without even knowing it. This means that you perspire at least a pint of sweat into your bedclothes each night. So the mattress and bedding need proper airing. A clammy bed offers you a poor welcome for good sleep. Most beds provide some way to let the air get at the underside of the mattress. This is the main reason why it is not a good idea to sleep on the floor: the bedding just does not get aired properly. Some Swiss believe that airing the bedding by hanging it out of the window in the alpine breezes and sunshine ensures a good night's sleep. Even if you have no alpine scenery or sunshine outside your bedroom window, it is easy to air your bed. Ten minutes with the covers pulled back in a warm room will do it. So launch your night's (or day's) sleep in a roomy, comfortable, warm, and well-aired bed; it's a good way to start the voyage.

Darken your sleeproom

Darkness has a natural and healthy link to sleep. We do not have the sensitive eyes of nighttime prowlers and pouncers like cats and owls. We humans are creatures of the day, and the sleep that we all need is firmly linked to the dark. Light is therefore an enemy of sleep, whether you are trying to get to sleep at night or during the day after a night of shift work. Here is how to deal with the sleeproom light problems you face as a shift worker.

1. Prevention is better than cure. Think about light pollution when choosing your house or apartment, picking your sleeproom, or selecting a motel, and try to get a sleeproom on the shady (north) side of the building. Blinds or curtains can help to keep out daylight, but aluminum foil taped to your sleeproom windows can give total darkness and will help keep your sleeproom cool. Foil reflects heat as well as light.

2. Dodge daylight. Shift work often involves trying to sleep during the day. Added to broken sleep routines and daytime noise, the power of sunlight can be a major problem. Recent sleep research has shown that for your body clock, daylight and darkness are the two most important regulators. This means that if you want to adapt to night shift, you must be like a mole in the morning; avoid daylight as much as you can. Get into your dark sleeproom as soon as possible.

3. Use an eyeshade mask. Made of soft black cloth with elastic to hold it in place, these inexpensive, simple masks deserve to be a lot more popular than they are. When you slip one on you have total darkness. Some airlines offer them to their passengers to help them sleep in the bright sunlight above the clouds. If you can't buy one, a strip of black velvet with a nose-notch cut in it and a safety pin closure will tide you over, but with a strip of elastic, needle and thread, anybody can make a mask in about five minutes. It's the kind of important detail that can make the difference between sleep and no sleep, especially if you are working shifts away from home.

Ventilate your sleeproom

The human lung is a masterpiece of plumbing. Each breath you take follows millions of branchings until it reaches the 400 million tiny air chambers on the surface of your lungs. In the delicate walls of these chambers, the blood supply, which also arrives there through millions of branchings, can exchange waste carbon dioxide for life-giving oxygen. To allow polluted air into this vital and delicate system is like mixing garbage with your food. Such abuse lowers your health at all times; it also means that you sleep less well.

Air pollution in the major cities where most people in America now live poses a major problem that is only slowly being tackled. But within each city, air pollution varies greatly from place to place. So you do have some control over how much garbage will go into your lungs and the lungs of your family. This means that when you are picking a place to live in the city, you should make air quality one of your prime goals. Here's how.

1. Avoid the polluters. Obviously, avoid factory chimneys, refineries, highways, and major traffic routes, but think also about prevailing winds and what they bring. The smoke from those tall chimneys pollutes a long way downwind. If you want to know what the prevailing or most common wind directions are in your city, get a map that shows how the airport runways are laid out. These runways are lined up with the most common wind directions to help shorten takeoff and landing runs. Phone the airport weather office if you are in doubt.

2. Head for the hills. Elevation is something else to think about, because air pollution is generally worst in low-lying areas. Wealthier suburbs of most cities are on high ground mainly for the view, but also for better air quality. So try to live higher up, even if the affordable housing has no view. Wherever you live, try to get a sleeproom above ground level. You will be glad, for instance, that your bedroom window is eight feet up on cold winter days when your neighbor leaves his car running for ten minutes to warm up, while its smoke drifts in a growing cloud at ground level. Or you might congratulate yourself for deciding to pay a little more for an apartment ten floors up when you look down at the clouds of blue traffic smoke below. Having picked the

best-air-quality neighborhood possible, you should think next about the air in your sleeproom.

During eight hours of sleep you will consume 130 cubic feet (3,600 liters) of air. That would fill a balloon six feet across! A 13 by 10 feet bedroom with an 8-foot high ceiling contains 1,040 cubic feet of this lifegiving gas. So after eight hours, two people in this sleeproom are breathing air that is one quarter stale, if there is no ventilation. Breathing stale air is no way to sleep well, so ventilate your sleeproom at all costs. If opening the window in daytime lets in noise, an open window in a nearby bathroom or another room can bring you fresh air.

So bring good air to your sleeproom by living in the least polluted part of the city and by proper sleeproom ventilation; your lungs deserve it, and better sleep will be one of your rewards.

Demand a quiet sleeproom

A lawn mower whining close to your window, a saw screaming its way through lumber, a vacuum cleaner growling and snarling overhead, a TV soap babbling at high volume in the apartment next to yours are among the noisy enemies of sleep. It may also be the neighbor's kids having noisy fun, their dog going for the Guinness nonstop-barking record, or their teenage son tuning his motorcycle and then doing circuits around the block. Any of these can be hell for a shift worker trying to sleep.

Some people can sleep through almost any noise. "What thunderstorm?" they ask their bleary-eyed companions at breakfast. But for most shift workers, sleep-wrecking noise, and especially daytime noise, is a major problem. Even noise that does not waken you, like the sounds of a refrigerator or an air conditioner, still takes its toll and lowers the quality of your sleep.

You probably must learn to sleep with some surrounding noise, but how perfect should you expect things to be? I think a good rule of thumb here is to be about as tolerant of imperfection as an army drill sergeant. Day or night, good sleep is your right! Anyone or anything that might deny you that right had better watch out.

So be feisty about any threats to your sleep, but like any smart fighter, be skilled at avoiding trouble. Prevention is better than cure (as with light problems). Here are several ways to avoid sleep-wrecking noises before they can give you trouble.

1. House hunt for quiet. When you go apartment or house hunting, search for a quiet neighborhood, a quiet street, and a quiet house. You may have found an area that you like on a weekend or holiday, when factories and freeways are not going full blast. Always visit the area on a weekday before making your final choice, or you may have some noisy surprises. You would also be smart to inquire at city hall about upcoming construction projects near to your possible home. A giant shopping plaza may be slated for the vacant block opposite, and it might soon be roaring with giant concrete trucks and all of the other daytime sleep-wrecking noises of construction.

   When you are house hunting, try to find one where daytime noise from children, washing machines, and the neighbor's lawn mower will be well away from your sleeproom. A house with a basement play space is a must if you have kids. Double-glazed windows are a big help. They insulate against sound as well as cold or heat. When checking out apartments, remember that your neighbors may be on all sides. A concrete apartment building will obviously be quieter than a wooden one. Remember, too, to avoid an apartment right next to the elevators, or one close to street level. It will be well worth the higher rent to be high up in the building where you will escape the noise (and smoke) of traffic.

2. Start with a friendly request: When you move into your new home, visit your neighbors and introduce yourself. Let them know that you work shifts and how much you will appreciate their consideration when you are trying to sleep in daylight hours. Get into the role of "good neighbor" and enjoy it. People naturally respond better to a friendly request for quiet from

a person who has pleasantly introduced themselves than to an angry complaint about noise from a red-faced stranger. You might even slip a card under their door as a reminder when you begin a series of night shifts and drop thank-you cards later if all goes well. Your cards might look something like these:

Hi Neighbor! My name is _____ and I have just moved in to_____. My job involves shift work, which means that I sometimes have to get my rest during the daytime. If you can avoid sleep-disturbing noise at these times:

Mon   Tues   Wed   Thur   Fri   Sat   Sun

Times:

you will have my sincere appreciation.

Thanks,

(your name goes here)

A GREAT BIG THANK YOU!!!!

for your thoughtfulness and courtesy in helping provide a noise-free neighborhood in which I can get my daytime rest. Thanks again!

Your neighbor,

(your name goes here)

You might let families with young children know that in an emergency their children can come to you as a block parent for help. In this way, you get to know your neighbors and present yourself as a good neighbor deserving respect and consideration.

3. There's still noise out there! You did the rounds and introduced yourself. You were surprised at how friendly and
sympathetic everyone was. But now, for the last two mornings when you were trying to sleep after exhausting graveyard shifts, a noisy neighbor kept you awake. Time to get
feisty? No. Time to take action? Certainly. If you have a good
personal relationship with them, phone or visit and remind
them how important quiet is for your sleep. Or you may
prefer to drop off a reminder card, something like this one:

Reminder

You will remember that my job involves shift work,
which means that I sometimes have to get my rest during
the daytime. I would very much appreciate if you can
avoid sleep-disturbing noise at these times:

          Mon   Tues   Wed   Thur   Fri   Sat   Sun

Times:

                                   Thanks again,
                                   Your neighbor

However annoying the noise has been, tell yourself that what
you are dealing with here is almost certainly thoughtlessness
and forgetfulness. Be patient.

4. THERE'S STILL NOISE OUT THERE! You have been
friendly and have let the neighbors know that you are a shift
worker, you have dropped off cards telling them when you
are on graveyard shift, you have dropped off three reminder
cards to a noisy neighbor, and there is STILL noise out there!
Time to get feisty? Definitely! Now you know that you are
dealing with a neighbor whose attitude is at best, "Who
cares?" and at worst, "To hell with you!" This is where your
patience and goodwill pays off. You have made all the right
moves and you have also kept track of dates and events. You

have put yourself in a strong position to make an effective complaint.

Complain to the apartment manager if you live in an apartment. Put your complaint in writing so that the manager knows how reasonable you have been and exactly what you are complaining about. Ninety-nine percent of apartment managers will act on a complaint presented like this. If you run into number 100, make it clear that your next written complaint will go to the apartment owners. As I said, get feisty.

If you live in a condo, you can bring it up at one of the regular meetings that condo owners have. Here again, the records that you have kept will show that your complaint is reasonable and valid.

If you live in a house and your noisy neighbor has resisted all reasonable approaches, it is time to contact the appropriate people at city hall. The department that you want may be named Environmental Health, Noise Control, Bylaw Enforcement, or Health Department. Keep up your search by phone until you have got an inspector on the line who handles noise complaints. This inspector may want something in writing from you, which is no problem. Your well-supported complaint will probably be taken seriously and acted on.

Finally, is it really worth spending so much time and trouble visiting neighbors, leaving notes, and so on, to get some peace and quiet? Yes it is—up to a point. Clearly, it's a trade-off. Think of the effort involved in getting neighbors to be considerate and helpful about your needs for peace and quiet. Obviously this effort should be a lot less than the effort of finding a new place and moving to it. Think of it as fine tuning your sleep situation. If, on the other hand, you find yourself involved in an exhausting ongoing war with neighbors about noise, then a well-researched move to a quieter area is indicated.

5. Hard-core city noise can be silenced too—up to a point: Far harder to deal with than these neighborhood noises are the noises of people going about their business. Traffic, trucks, buses, and trains all run late into the night in most big cities, as well as going full blast all day. Police and fire engine sirens scream, jets roar overhead. What can you do about these? The answer is fight-or-flight.

If you are prepared to fight, don't try to fight alone. If local noise bothers you, it probably bothers a lot of other people too. They may already have formed a group to put pressure on city hall. So find them and consider joining them. Such groups are often successful in getting noise bylaws or zoning laws changed or enforced. Even the knowledge that you are fighting back will help to make a noise more bearable. But while you may have some important local successes by fighting back, you can't expect to shut down New York. The core areas of most big cities are really not fit to live in, with their heavy noise and air pollution from traffic. This pollution damages not only your sleep, but also your waking hours. So if this is your situation, like millions before you, you should consider a move to somewhere cleaner and quieter. In other words, when it no longer makes sense to fight, then flight may be the smart solution.

That pretty well takes care of the noises outside your sleeproom; let's finish with the noises inside it.

1. Tame your telephone. By far the commonest noisemaker that people tolerate in their sleeprooms is the telephone. Making calls to a soothing friend from your sleeproom just before going to sleep makes sense, and having the thing there so that you can summon the police or fire department gives peace of mind. But unless your job involves being on-call, muzzle it. Switch off the bell. Otherwise you give every telephone in the world the right to disturb your sleep! And if you are female and living alone, your bedside phone is open to calls from

anonymous weirdos; that's no way to get good sleep. You may also get junk calls, telephone solicitations business that can wait, and wrong numbers. Also, some bosses think they have the right to call you at any hour of the day or night. Don't let them. Put an answering machine on the living room phone, record a courteous message on it, and have a good sleep. Do not be a slave to your phone.

2. Subdue your air conditioner. Air conditioners are the loudest noisemakers that most people tolerate in the sleeproom. I have worked out of motels in the desert country of California and Arizona in June and July, and I am familiar with every clatter, gurgle, hum, and whirr that these monsters can make. The heat has to be pretty bad before I will switch one on. I found that quite a good routine for night sleep is to have the thing going full blast all evening while I am out, and then switch it off and open a window before going to sleep. Ideally, the hotel or motel will have one big air conditioner far from your sleeproom, rather than one of these noisemakers per room. It is something to watch for when picking a motel in the hot country.

If you absolutely must have an air conditioner in your own sleeproom, check the sound level before purchasing it.

Other minor noises in the bedroom come from noisy clocks (replace them with a digital one) and energetic pets (shut them out).

Finally, what can you do right now about inescapable noise, like traffic noise? I suggest putting a pillow on top of your head as well as below it. It can work pretty well for tonight. Tomorrow go and buy a large (3-foot) down-filled pillow. When you are ready to sleep, shake and squeeze it in the middle until it has an hourglass shape, and then sleep with it wrapped around your head with only your face showing. I have slept like this for years and highly recommend it. When you travel, take it with you. Down pillows are very light and can be squeezed into a small space. You may prefer ear plugs, which are available at any drugstore, but don't plug your ears so thoroughly that you can not be woken by a smoke alarm.

Keep personal and world troubles out of your sleeproom

Personal and world troubles do not belong in your sleeproom. Here is how to keep them out.

1. Keep out personal troubles. Try and keep all talk of personal troubles out of your sleeproom. This is not always easy. Very often couples want to talk or argue about problems in privacy, and the sleeproom is the most convenient place to do it. Also, it is quite natural for the past day's, or tomorrow's, troubles to come to your mind just before you sleep. It may be difficult to keep out problems, troubles, arguments, and squabbles, but it can be done quite simply: just decide that they are not appropriate in your sleeproom. You make decisions of this kind very often. For instance, you decide that it is not appropriate to quarrel in front of guests or in the workplace. There is nearly always some other room in the house where a couple can discuss, dispute, or fight over their differences. It is often a good idea to take a walk or drive somewhere to argue on neutral ground. A car is a very private place. The point is this: it is worth making the effort to link your sleeproom with peaceful and loving relations with your partner. Settle all differences with your partner outside the sleeproom, or postpone them. Enter the sleeproom only in a spirit of love and goodwill. You take your muddy boots off at the front door of your house to help keep your house clean. Respect the peace of your sleeproom in the same way.

2. Keep out the world's troubles. This is much easier. I am a worrywart when it comes to the world's troubles. Pollution, wars, highway accidents—I keep track of them all. But my wife and I have a strict rule: the world's troubles do not come into our sleeproom. We do not talk about these things, and try to avoid even thinking about them in there. This rule is stated

very well in the movie classic *Cabaret* by the German emcee of the cabaret (Joel Grey): "Leave your troubles outside. Zo! Life is disappointing? Forget it! Inside here everything is beautiful." Keeping troubles outside is an important part of turning your bedroom into a beautiful sleeproom.

Get rid of haunting memories

Of all the rooms in a house, the sleeproom is the most likely to be haunted. This is mainly because it is the room that we occupy when we are most alone with our thoughts and memories. Memories of great happiness or sadness are more likely to haunt us here—especially in the middle of the night—than in any other room. Here are some ways to banish these ghosts that keep us awake.

1. Change the furniture: Change the room as much as possible. Move the bed to a new location, or get a new one; paint the walls a new color; change the lighting; hang new pictures. Change your bedtime routines (see Chapter 4). In fact, do all that you can to make your new sleeproom as unlike the old one as possible. Break as many of the links with the past as you can.

2. Change the atmosphere. To remove problem ghosts, have a housewarming party. The purpose of any housewarming party is to have your friends in to link a new place to the good people in your life. It doesn't matter how long you have lived where you are. Throw a housewarming party. Ghosts tend to drift away when the good times roll.

Create a secure sleeproom

Your sleeproom must be a refuge where you can go to escape from the world and all its troubles. This sometimes means locking the door to keep people out. It also means taking steps to safeguard against the most threatening of all intruders—smoke and fire. Here is how to have a secure sleeproom.

1. Bolts and chains. In your own home you will probably leave your sleeproom unlocked and depend on the front door, which should be securely locked, to keep out intruders. The only reason for a lock on the sleeproom door is so that mom and dad can have some privacy.

   In many apartments, the door to your sleeproom is your front door. Depending on this door lock is not good enough. Management does not change the lock every time a departing tenant fails to return the keys. Bolting and chaining these doors is not paranoid; it's smart.

2. Fire prevention. A secure sleep room involves much more than keeping out intruders. It involves the security of the entire building in which you are sleeping. When you sleep you are at your most helpless. The strongest man in the world, while sleeping, can be overcome by a child with a box of matches. If the building in which you are sleeping is built of wood, has no smoke detectors, has a cluttered messy basement where paint, oil, rags, and newspapers are stored, has electrical extension cords snaking in all directions, has a garage built into the basement, and has one or more smokers puffing away, then you live in a firetrap. Even if only two or three of these fire hazards exist in your home, they may be quietly preying on your mind and making it hard for you to get to sleep (they *should* be making it hard for you to get to sleep). So fix them, and most important, install and maintain smoke detectors. Fires and smoke kill about five thousand Americans a year. Removing the risks of being one of them will make it easier for you to go to sleep.

So the kind of security that will help turn your bedroom into a sleeproom comes after you have dealt with real and probable threats such as smoke, fire, and intruders. Security and peace of mind come from knowing that these problems are taken care of as much as is reasonably possible.

How to choose a hotel or motel sleeproom

Many shift workers' jobs take them far from home. Next time you rent a motel or hotel room, make sure that you are getting a sleeproom. Here is a checklist to help you make a good choice:

1. Check the motel/hotel:

   ■ Phone ahead. Reserve ahead if you can, and pick a motel chain that you know.

   ■ Building construction. Concrete is best. Wooden multi-unit buildings let you hear your neighbor's TV, and they also burn better than concrete.

   ■ Security. Is the building fitted with smoke alarms and sprinklers? (There has never been a fire death to date in any building properly fitted with sprinklers in the United States.)

   ■ Noise. How close are heavy traffic, railroads, major construction projects, or industry? Can they give you a room far from elevators, bars, restaurants, kitchens, and alleys where noisy deliveries are made at all hours?

   ■ Is there a main air conditioner, or is there one of these noisy monsters per room?

2. Check out the room. When you arrive at the desk, always ask to see the room before checking in. The five-minute delay involved is well worth it. It can save you an uncomfortable night or the inconvenience of changing rooms later on when there are fewer vacancies. Here is what to look for in your potential sleeproom:

   ■ Ventilation: Is the air fresh, or is it musty, damp, or tainted by tobacco-smoke-drenched furnishings?

   ■ Temperature: Is it comfortable, stifling hot or chilly cold? Does the air conditioner work, and is it quiet? How is the room heated, and where is the thermostat?

■ The bed: Is it comfortable? Is it bone dry? (Slip your hand between the sheets and you may get a clammy surprise, as I did in one poorly heated motel.) Are there enough covers and extra blankets in the closet?

■ Noise: Is the room truly as quiet as the desk claimed? Is there a parking lot outside that will be noisy later on when the bar is in full swing? Can you hear any TV sounds through thin walls when you walk through the corridors?

■ Security: You need peace of mind and a feeling of security to sleep well in a strange place. Are you secure from fire and smoke? Are there sprinklers, smoke detectors, fire doors, and well-marked fire escapes? If you are in a multistory hotel, is the stairway that exits to the roof clearly marked? In the fire at the MGM Grand in Las Vegas, some guests were forced by smoke to climb to the top of one stairway and were trapped there; the other stairway led to a roof exit and helicopter rescue. Does the door have a secure bolt and chain? The key, remember, provides little security.

It takes little time to do this kind of inspection to make sure that you have a comfortable, secure sleeproom, and it is well worth it. The payoff is a good restful sleep.

Welcome to your sleeproom

You have by now transformed your bedroom into a sleeproom. All links to daytime activities, such as your sewing machine, your computer, your suitcases, and your skis, have gone. Everything in this room is now linked to sleep. A comfortable bed waits in a well-ventilated, quiet, secure, and beautiful room that is a refuge from the world. Walking into it, talking about it, even thinking about it should make you feel drowsy and have you yawning. Welcome to your . . . (Yawn) . . . Sleeproom.

4

Food, exercise, and sex
for good sleep

Gary, a friend of mine, loves dogs but thinks that it would be cruel to keep one in his city apartment. "It wouldn't get enough exercise and fresh air," he says regretfully. Yet Gary lives in an apartment, and at 190 pounds, he is bigger than any dog. He smokes, drinks, and gets no more exercise than walking to his car or to the corner store. Gary would never give a dog the fried meats or highly spiced food that he often eats for dinner himself. To give a dog several ounces of ethyl alcohol, a notorious nerve poison, would not occur to him. Yet Gary often downs a double scotch on the rocks. Gary, in fact, treats himself much worse than he would treat a dog. His poor health, his lackluster love life, and his sleep problems are therefore not surprising.

People like Gary are becoming more rare these days. Fitness is fashionable, and people are learning that being "kind to your body" enormously improves not only the soundness of your sleep, but the overall quality of your life (including your sex life).

Fitness is especially important for you as a shift worker. Shift work tends to take some of the quality out of your life and your sleep by upsetting your life schedules. This chapter will help you restore some of that quality by suggesting ways to improve your diet, your exercise, and your sex life. One of your many rewards will be better sleep.

Food and better sleep

One of the many revolutions in America in the last twenty years has been the food revolution. Americans today have much healthier eating habits than in the past. This shows in our speech: expressions such as "low cholesterol," "high fiber," "organic vegetables," "no additives," and "junk food" have all become part of our language and thinking. The marketplace has not been slow to adapt to this change, and tasty health foods are now widely featured in cookbooks and restaurants. The trend towards healthier eating seems to be here to stay.

What is the connection between health food and sleep? Apart from the long-term health benefits to your digestive tract, heart, and arteries, there is an important immediate effect: health food is easier to digest than the old staples such as cheeseburgers, steak, pork chops, and roast beef.

When you rest, all of you should rest—including your stomach. Do not expect your stomach to let you have a good sleep if you have given it heavy work to do. The heaviest work for your stomach is digesting fatty foods. A large meal of roast beef, gravy, fries, and cheesecake will keep your stomach busy for about eight hours. You will not sleep soundly while this work is in progress. In contrast, a meal of grilled fish and vegetables is a light digestion job, which your stomach will finish in about an hour. This does not mean that you can never have roast beef for dinner again. It does mean that if you want to sleep well, go easy on the fats and treat your stomach with respect.

In general, eat:

1. Salads of all kinds, but avoid rich, oily salad dressings.

2. Seafoods of all kinds, especially steamed, grilled, or lightly fried.

3. White meat such as chicken and turkey.

4. Vegetables of all kinds, boiled, steamed, microwaved, or raw.

5. Pasta of all kinds, but avoid the heavy meat sauces.

6. Fresh fruit.

7. Small helpings.

In general, avoid:

1. Fried foods of all sorts, including those fried in batter.

2. Red meats such as beef, pork, and veal, especially when they are fried or roasted and smothered in gravy.

3. Heavy, spicy cheese dishes such as lasagna.

4. Rich desserts with icing and whipping cream.

5. Alcohol and coffee.

6. Large helpings or seconds.

7. Food-vending machines and 24-hour fast-food chains.

Exercise and better sleep

If you had to load "Sixteen Tons" of coal by hand, working in a mine, lack of exercise would not be one of your problems. But the days of heavy physical shift work are long gone. Human muscle is now one of the most expensive forms of power, so management avoids using it as much as possible; it's much cheaper to use machines. Exercise on the job is now rare.

But even when you leave your job, the machines are all around waiting to do work for you: automobiles, lawn mowers, washing machines, elevators, escalators, power tools—the variety of machines that have replaced muscle is almost endless. They have replaced much drudgery and monotonous work, which is great. But they may be killing you with kindness. The automobile probably kills more people by denying them exercise than it does in accidents.

The replacement of muscle by machines means that you are unlikely to get enough healthy exercise in a typical day on the job and around home. Exercise no longer comes to you. You have to get up and go chase it; you have to decide to exercise.

If you have trouble making this decision and sticking with it, it may help to ask the "why" question about exercise. I once asked a seventy-three-year-old geologist named Max Martin why he exercised so hard.

Max and I were working on a drill job on a silver prospect in the eastern California desert. It was scorching hot. In the blazing desert sun, Max would carry the fifty-pound core boxes two hundred yards uphill from the drill rig, although we had a truck to do the job. He would jump out of the truck to clear rocks off the old dirt road we traveled daily. He dragged an eight-foot long eight-by-eight timber several hundred feet and made a ladder out of it to get down an old shaft. At other times he would be out all day in the desert prospecting with only a few cans of V-8 juice in his pack. He was always looking for physical work to do. He was thin as a rake and hard as nails.

"Max," I said, "you're a glutton for exercise. How come?"

"The more I exercise the better I feel," he answered. He said nothing about losing weight, living longer, looking trim, improving his sex life and his cardiovascular system, or sleeping better, although all of these benefits come from exercise. "Feeling better" said it all for him.

Ask children why they like to run, skip, jump, hop, swim, and play games. "It's fun!" will almost certainly be the answer in some form or other.

Watch dancers, skaters, swimmers, and athletes and see the joy they get out of moving their bodies.

"Feeling better," "fun," the joy of movement—these are the positive, here-and-now answers to the "why" question. If you are getting pleasure out of exercise and its results, you will keep doing it; if it is a chore or a duty, you will find reasons to quit. So how you think about exercise and your attitude towards it can put muscle in your decision to start.

Once you have decided that you want to exercise, like Max, you may start looking for exercise anywhere you can find it. His attitude certainly inspired me. If the phone rings now, I jump up and get it.

My wife wants a glass of juice? I'm in the kitchen right now pouring it. Garden needs digging? Garbage to go out? It's done. By nature I'm lazy, but I have now got into the habit of enjoying exercise. Of course, jumping up to answer the phone is pretty skimpy exercise. The most important muscle to exercise is the one you never see—your heart.

It took a bit of a scare to get me interested in heart exercises. Back in August 1970 I had the job of looking at a copper prospect on a steep mountainside in British Columbia. The nearby town of Lytton often sets high-temperature records for Canada. I had climbed about 1,500 feet up the mountain in a temperature between ninety and one hundred, and was so exhausted I had to lie down and sleep for about two hours. The next day it was a little easier, and on the third day I was in fairly good shape again. When I got home I vowed I would never get out of condition like that again, and I started jogging every morning. Twenty-four years later I am still jogging daily.

Jogging is a widely approved form of cardiovascular or heart exercise. The beauty of it is that you are completely in charge. You can slow down or quit any time you feel uncomfortable, unlike in some competitive or team sports where you may be pressured by other players to overexert. I always enjoy jogging. I enjoy the fresh morning air; I say "Good morning" to everyone I meet; if it is raining I carry an umbrella. On the rare occasions when I am not enjoying it, I quit. That way, it has never become a duty or a chore.

Jogging tends to suit shift workers. You are free to schedule it whenever you want—a big advantage over gyms, tennis courts, and swimming pools. Also, the clothing and equipment needed are very simple. You can start jogging now without buying anything or paying fees to anyone. Security can be a problem in jogging, especially for women. The answer is to find a safe and beautiful place to jog, even if you have to drive ten or fifteen minutes to get there. If that is not practical, you can jog at home on a treadmill or ride a bicycling machine.

Many exercises besides jogging can give your heart a good workout, for example, swimming, bicycling, cross-country skiing, and tennis. All of these exercises can give your heart the sustained work it needs at your "training heart rate." Your training heart rate is your own redline heart rate when you are exercising. Here is how to figure it out:

1. Subtract your age from 220; this will give you your maximum heart rate.

2. 60% of your maximum heart rate is your training heart rate. (If you are using a simple calculator, just multiply your maximum heart rate by 0.6 to get your training heart rate.)

Here are some examples:

Age	Maximum Heart Rate	Training Heart Rate
30	220-30 = 190	60% of 190 = 114
40	220-40 = 180	60% of 180 = 108
50	220-50 = 170	60% of 170 = 102

This table shows that if you are fifty years old, your heart rate should not go above 102 beats per minute when you are exercising.

Your heart exercise is the most important one for you to do. But once you are rolling, you may wish to explore other forms of exercise, those that get you involved with other people and those that help you learn and practice new skills.

Social exercises give you the chance to meet, be with, or enjoy the company of other people while you exercise. Moving to music with well-shaped members of the opposite sex in trendy skintight clothing can be a pleasant way to develop your body and your social life. Fitness and health club listings filling many columns in the Yellow Pages, show how popular social exercise has become.

Skill development exercises allow you to develop athletic skills while exercising. The variety is enormous and many of the activities are also social. The distinction is that here your priority is skill development rather than social interaction. You might want to develop skill in dancing, martial arts, tennis, skating, volleyball, baseball—the list goes on.

The timing of your exercise is important. For your heart exercise, one of the best times is shortly after you get up. Less strenuous exercise can be done at any time except in the hour or two before you wish to sleep. You may find that shift work gives you some exercise advantages in the form of less-crowded sport facilities during the day.

Finally, finding the time for exercise may not be easy, especially if you are on irregular shifts. Many shift work jobs can be so exhausting that days off are taken up largely by sleep and recovery. However part of the health benefit of exercise is the extra energy and alertness that it gives. It is a very tight daily schedule that does not have twenty minutes somewhere for a jog and a shower.

Sex and better sleep

Your sex life, which is such an important part of your love life, can be threatened by shift work. This is intolerable. No job is worth a threatened or broken marriage or the loss of a loved partner. Shift work's threats to your love life must be tackled head-on and solved. The main threat comes from shift work scheduling and its effects.

Shift work tends to upset your sex schedules just as it upsets your sleep and digestive schedules. You can solve your sleep and digestion schedule problems alone but you need your partner's cooperation to solve your sex schedule problem. Here are some issues to consider in talking this over with your partner.

1. Priority. How important is sex in your relationship? If the answer is "very," or "central," then you will probably not be willing to put it off until the weekend or shift change. You will not squeeze it into a corner of leftover time. You will likely decide that your sex life must always get prime time, whatever shift you are on. Football and baseball, sitcoms, and TV specials can all wait. Your dignity as a human being demands that your sex life get priority.

2. Prime time. The best time for sex is when you are both rested and feel like lovemaking. Such times are scarcer for shift workers than for those on day shifts and are therefore more

valuable. They may happen during the day or in the evening when the children are active and demanding. Baby-sitters may be inconvenient or costly, but compared to the emotional trauma and inconvenience of breakups and the costs of divorce courts and lawyers, the expense is trifling. Pay it gladly.

3. Scheduling. If your partner is free during the day and you are working evening or night shifts, you have no problem scheduling your sex life. But these days in 57 percent of U.S. families, both parents work. If your partner works the same shifts as you, there's no problem; it is when your partner works days, for instance, that your lives, including your sex lives, can get out of sync. You may want to sit down together and agree on your prime times for sex. When you work shifts you have to plan time "nests" just like you prepare a love nest. Enjoy it. You can make "dates," and the anticipation will certainly brighten up your shift and your partner's lonely evenings and nights.

4. Fatigue. Shift workers do not sleep as well as day workers. That is why this book is in your hands. If loss of interest in sex, due to fatigue, is a problem for you, then what you are finding here may help you. Your partner's love and understanding and your own frankness and willingness to talk things over can help you through the rough spots.

5. Talk. Sex is an area where people can be very vulnerable to feelings of inadequacy or rejection. Talking about a sexual relationship is not always easy. At one extreme are couples who criticize, psychologize, rationalize, and talk it all to death. If sex life is compared to a forest, this couple wants to clear-cut it and remove all mystery. At the other extreme are couples who say nothing and depend on instinct and telepathy; this couple may easily lose track of each other in the sexual "forest." A happy medium is the couple who have cut out trails of love and understanding in this sexual forest, but who are content to leave large areas of mystery.

6. Sex and sleep: Good sleep nearly always follows good sex. Nobody needs to have this proved to them by scientific studies. The other side of this coin, of course, is that troubled sex leads to troubled sleep. If shift work is the source of this trouble, then, as mentioned earlier, meet the trouble head-on. Don't delay or avoid it. This is not a part of your life that you should yield to anything. If shift work keeps threatening your sex life in spite of all your efforts, then it may be time to consider this question: Are the benefits that you get from shift work so great that they outweigh your sex and love life?

Step 4

Take a Hard Look
at the Drugs in Your Life

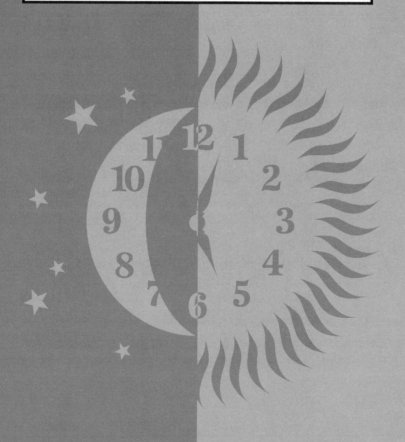

5

Sleeping pills
can be a pact with the devil

Sleeping pills and their relatives, the tranquilizers, are the most heavily prescribed drugs in the United States. Between 6 and 9 million adults annually consume 630 million sleeping pills. Each of these pills weighs about one gram, so the total weight consumed in a year in the U.S. is 695 tons! That's one hundred and thirty-nine five-ton dump trucks full.

Yet most sleeping pills give abnormal sleep and worsen the user's ability to function. No sleeping pill is effective for longer than one month, according to the *American Medical Association Guide to Better Sleep*. Also, most sleeping pills are habit-forming and if used for longer than two or three weeks may cause difficult to severe withdrawal effects. They thus offer short-term gain for long-term pain, a kind of "pact with the devil."

"Sleeping pills are presently overprescribed and overused," writes Dr. E. Hartmann, a professor of psychiatry at Tufts University School of Medicine in Boston and director of the Sleep-Dream Laboratory at Boston State Hospital. "As sleeping pills are being used now, my conclusion is that the overall risks outweigh the overall benefits . . . Currently prescribed hypnotics are mostly non-specific CNS (brain and spinal cord) depressants whose mode of action has nothing to do with the normal biology of sleep."

What are sleeping pills?

Obviously a sleeping pill is a pill that makes you sleep or makes you sleepy. It may be a drug in the form of a pill, a liquid, or a capsule. Not so obviously, it may be an alcohol "night cap," it may be an antihistamine, or it may be a tranquilizer.

If you had lived in London one hundred years ago you might have used Dalby's Carminative, Godfrey's Cordial, or Dover's Powder to help yourself sleep, and to help the children sleep you might have used Winslow's Soothing Syrup or Street's Infant Quietness. All of these sleeping potions from the last century contained opium. This casual use of opium would be shocking today but was normal and widely accepted back then. Opium has many disadvantages as a sleeping pill, the chief ones being that it is highly addictive and has very severe withdrawal effects.

Chloral hydrate was used increasingly as a sleeping pill following its synthesis in 1832 and remains in use today. Its effect weakens with use as tolerance develops, and the sleep that it brings is abnormal, with less REM and deep sleep.

Barbiturates first appeared in 1911. Eventually over fifty types were marketed, although only about three are commonly used now. They rapidly became the main ingredient in the world's sleeping pills, in spite of the dangerously small difference between a dose and an overdose.

The benzodiazepine group of drugs appeared in the early 1960s. The drugs Dalmane, Halcion, Valium, and Librium belong to this group, which has largely replaced the barbiturates in the sleeping pill and tranquilizer market. The great advantage that this sleep inducing and tranquilizing group of drugs had over barbiturates was that they were much safer. The difference between a dose and an overdose for these drugs is large. However, the sleep that these drugs bring is not normal; their use can cause physical dependency and withdrawal symptoms; taken with alcohol they can be dangerous. The search for an ideal sleeping pill goes on.

So what is an ideal sleeping pill? Many doctors agree that it should at least satisfy these four essentials:

1. Safety. How safe are the pills if you happen to take more than the prescribed dose? It can happen by accident, for instance, to someone who wakes up and forgets having already taken a pill, and sleepily takes two more. Also, sleeping pills are often prescribed for people suffering from depression. It is obviously unsafe for such people to have a bottle of sleeping pills, which can become suicide pills by merely increasing the dose. With some barbiturates, just ten times the prescribed dose can be harmful. How safe are the pills in combination with other prescribed medications or with alcohol? Some of these combinations interact to be harmful.

2. Sleep. The ideal pill will bring sleep with little delay. This sleep should be a normal sleep with all of the usual mix of shallow, deep, and REM sleep that makes up the normal ninety-minute sleep cycle. The sleeper should wake up after eight hours of uninterrupted sleep feeling refreshed. When the ideal pill is discontinued, even after being used for weeks or months, sleep remains normal. The ideal pill will also be specific for sleep; in other words, its only effect will be to induce and maintain sleep. It will not be a "shotgun" medication that hits the sleep target and many other bodily function targets as well in an uncomfortable, or even damaging, spray of side effects.

3. Hangover. The effects of the ideal pill will stop after eight hours so that the sleeper can wake up fully alert, relaxed, and clearheaded and with absolutely no hangover. Ability to drive a car in traffic, pilot a plane, or perform brain surgery should be quite unaffected by the sleeping pill taken eight hours before. Those leading less active lives, such as seniors, also have the right to expect a sleeping pill to leave them relaxed and clearheaded the next morning.

4. Addiction. The ideal pill is one that gives good sleep, time after time, without the need to increase the dose. Also, when users stop taking this ideal pill, even after weeks of use, there

are no bad effects of withdrawal, which may drive the users back to the pill for relief and thus make them addicted to it.

With these desirable features of the ideal sleeping pill fresh in your mind, take a look at the table on the following page, which shows some of the important features of all of the sleep-inducing drugs, or hypnotics.

Drugs	Safety (Overdose, dangerous interactions)	Sleep	Hangover (Fitness next day to drive, fly, and use machines)	Addictive (Tolerance with use. Withdrawal effects)
Opiates (Opium, morphine, heroin)	Danger of overdose, esp. with quinine and alcohol.	Abnormal: less REM and deep (stage 4) sleep.	Fitness affected.	Highly addictive. Tolerance increases with use. Withdrawal very severe.
Alcohol	Danger of overdose, especially with narcotics.	Abnormal: less REM.	Fitness affected.	Addictive. Tolerance increases. Withdrawal severe.
Chloral Hydrate (Noctec Aqua-chloral)	Use with alcohol causes heavy, to dangerous, sedation.	Abnormal: less REM and deep sleep.	Fitness affected.	Habit-forming. Tolerance in 2 weeks. With-drawal varies with dose.
Barbiturates (Luminal, Nembutal, Seconal, Amytal, etc.)	Major danger of overdose esp. with alcohol and narcotics.	Abnormal: less REM and deep (stages 3 and 4) sleep.	Fitness affected.	Addictive. Tolerance increases rapidly with use. Heavy use withdrawal very severe.
Benzodiazepines (Dalmane, Restoril, Halcion, and tranquilizers like Valium, Tranxene, and Librium.)	Safe, but use with alcohol causes heavy, to dangerous, sedation.	Abnormal: less REM and deep (stage 4) sleep.	Fitness affected (except for Restoril and Halcion).	Tolerance develops slowly. Very high dose withdrawal is severe. Low dose withdrawal after long use is difficult.
Diphenhydramine OTC Non Rx (Nytol with DPH, Sominex 2)	Use with alcohol causes excess sedation.	A mild sedative, depressed REM and deep (stage 4) sleep.	Fitness affected.	No data.
Melatonin	Safe, but long-term effects unknown.	Can reset sleep cycles.	Fitness not affected.	Not yet known to be habit forming.

This table gives only a crude picture of a complicated scene where you cannot afford to make mistakes. The information it gives is partly historical, since opium and barbiturates are no longer used as sleeping pills. Use it as a rough guide only. The troublesome to dangerous interactions of various drugs is a major study in itself.

A closer look at the most commonly used sleeping pills

The safest, the most trouble-free, the most effective, and therefore the most commonly used sleeping pills now are the benzodiazepine group. Since this group is so widely used and so important, you may want to know more about them. Here are the names of commonly used benzodiazepine sleeping pills.

Generic Name	Trade Names
Flurazepam:	Benozil, Dalmane, Dalmadorm, Dalmate, Domodor, Dormodor, Felison, Felmane, Flunox, Fordrim, Insumin, Lunipax, Midorm AR, Natam, Niotal, Remdue, Somlan, Valdorm
Loprazolam	Avlane, Dormonoct
Lormetazepam	Loramet, Noctamid
Nitrazepam	Apodorm, Arem, Benzalin, Calsmin, Dormicum, Dumolid, Eatan, Eunoctin, Hypsal, Hypnotin, Mitidin, Mogadan, Mogadon, Nelbon, Neuchlonic, Nipam, Nitrados, Nitrenpax, Noctene, Pacisyn, Paxisyn, Pelson, Persopir, Prosonno, Quill, Radedorm, Relact, Remnos, Sindepres, Somnased, Somnibel, Somnite, Sonebon, Sonnolin, Surem, Unisomnia
Temazepam	Cerepax, Euhypnos, Lenal, Levanxene, Levanxol, Mabertin, Maeva, Normison, Planum, Remestan, Restoril, Signopam
Triazolam	Halcion

This group of hypnotic, or sleep-inducing, drugs is so widely used and so important that it deserves a closer look. Here is how these sleeping pills measure up in detail if you ask the same questions that are asked in the table.

1. Safety. The safety of benzodiazepines is one of the key qualities that account for their popularity and domination of the sleeping pill market. Unlike barbiturates, benzodiazepines are not dangerous drugs. According to W. A. McKim, in *Drugs and Behavior*:

   "The outcomes of benzodiazepine overdose are virtually never fatal . . . There is no deep coma or severe respiratory depression . . . Most symptoms disappear within 48 hours."

   However, it is very important to remember, as McKim points out, when combined with alcohol these drugs, as well as many others, can be dangerous or even fatal.

2. Sleep quality. The quality of sleep assisted by benzodiazepine sleeping pills is, in general, lower than that of normal healthy sleep. However, there may be quite wide variations in sleep quality between individuals due to state of health, size of dose, age, length of treatment, and the type of benzodiazepine used. The most important negative effects are that essential deep sleep and REM sleep are both reduced by these drugs.

   "[These] hypnotics suppress both deep sleep and dreaming sleep (REMS) and the extra sleeping time is largely made up of a relatively light sleep . . . With rapidly eliminated benzodiazepines (eg, triazolam) there may be a rebound of dreaming sleep, sometimes accompanied by nightmares in the later part of the night."

   Note: Halcion (Triazolam), the world's most widely prescribed sleeping pill, was withdrawn from the U.K. market on October 2, 1991, by the British government's Department of Health on the recommendation of its Committee on the Safety of Medicines, which stated:

"It is now considered the risks of treatment with triazolam outweigh the benefits."

3. Hangover: After taking a benzodiazepine sleeping pill, how is your fitness the next day affected when it comes to driving a vehicle, piloting a plane, operating machinery, or doing any job demanding concentration and skill?

   The hangover effects of benzodiazepine sleeping pills largely depend on how rapidly your body can get rid of these drugs. The figure used to describe this is the "elimination half-life." The elimination half-life for nitrazepam is between fifteen and thirty-eight hours. This means that if you used a nitrazepam sleeping pill to get to sleep at 11:00 P.M. on Monday night, half of the dose that you took would still be active in your system until at least fifteen hours later, at 2:00 P.M. on Tuesday. However, depending on your health and age and the dose taken, it might take your body as long as thirty-eight hours to reduce the amount present in your system to half. In other words, the effects of the drug might last until 1:00 P.M. on Wednesday. H. Ashton wrote in a 1994 article for *Drugs*:

   "Nitrazepam commonly produces a subjective feeling of hangover and impairs performance the next day in single or repeated doses although subjective effects may decrease as tolerance develops."

   You can expect lesser hangover effects from benzodiazepine sleeping pills that are more rapidly eliminated. Here are three, with their elimination half-lives in hours: Loprazolam (6–12), Lormetazepam (10–12) and Temazepam (8–15).

4. Addiction: Benzodiazepine sleeping pills are not considered addictive. However, it is important to know that taking these pills for longer than a week or two often has penalties. Within just a few weeks, they lose their effectiveness in bringing sleep, and your sleep problems return as before. If you then stop taking these pills, you may have a rebound of the REM

sleep that these pills have been suppressing, and there may be other unpleasant withdrawal symptoms, including anxiety. The longer you have been taking the pills, the longer will the rebound and other symptoms last. This can lead some people to return to using the pills, not because of the wonderful sleep they bring, but just to avoid the unpleasant effects of withdrawal. It is not hard to see how this can become a vicious spiral of dependency.

Obviously no ideal sleeping pill exists, even among the benzodiazepines. As the tables show, they all have important drawbacks. These drawbacks range from serious or life-threatening ones (opium and barbiturates) to uncomfortable withdrawal effects on quitting after several weeks of use (benzodiazepines). Although some patients benefit from long-term use of sleeping pills, most shift workers should avoid them except for short-term emergency use.

Melatonin: magic sleeping pill?

Courier services take pride in rapidly delivering packages to exactly the right destination. Your body also has a courier service—your blood stream—which delivers chemical messages sent out by glands. These messages are called hormones, and they have exact chemical addresses, which are to-whom-it-may-concern types of messages. Adrenaline is a hormone; so is melatonin.

Melatonin is a hormone sent out from the pineal gland. Its best knows "address" is:

> To: Sleep center
> Suprachiasmatic Nucleus,
> Brain

When melatonin is delivered by your bloodstream to the suprachiasmatic nucleus, or sleep-center it sets the body-clock and tells it that now is a good time for sleep.

Although melatonin was discovered in 1958, it is only in the last few years that there has been much research into its effects. Many claims have been made for this hormone, which unlike the benzodiazepine sleeping pills, is easily available in health food stores.

Although claims have been made that melatonin supplements can improve sex life, arrest aging, cure cancer and bring sleep, the only effect that has been confirmed by widely accepted scientific experiments, is that melatonin can help reset the body clock.

Melatonin appears to be harmless, even when taken in large quantities, but its long term effects are not known. "Human hormones are powerful substances and can produce unexpected results in long-term use, or even in single large doses," says the *Berkeley Wellness Letter* of April 1995. "The long-term effects of melatonin on women is totally unexplored territory right now," says David Oren of the National Institute of Mental Health, quoted in *Health*, September 1995.

These warnings should be remembered, especially by people who are currently dosing themselves with very large amounts of melatonin. A healthy young adult produces about 0.03 mg of melatonin in 24 hours. Compare this with the amount of melatonin in pills currently available:

Melatonin "supplements" available	Equivalent to amount produced by your body during:
0.75 mg	25 days
2.0 mg	66 days
3.0 mg	100 days
5.0 mg	166 days
10.0 mg	333 days

The typical dose recommended on melatonin sold in health food stores is 3.0 mg. This, then, amounts to your body's melatonin production for 100 days or 3 months. That is a big dose of a relatively unknown hormone to pop into your mouth in one pill. It is also important to remember that the purity and potency of the melatonin sold in health food stores is not regulated.

So what to do? Obviously, melatonin is a hot item in the market. In November 1995, *Newsweek* reported " . . . The huge GNC chain, which didn't even carry melatonin until early September, was moving 4,000 bottles a day by the middle of the month." The health food stores are making money and want you to believe that melatonin is safe; the big drug companies want to move into the market with a refined, regulated, and certainly more costly product. Britain's Medicine Control Agency has halted the sale of melatonin until clinical tests prove its safety. But were they nudged by the big drug companies?

Glowing claims about melatonin conflict with dark warnings. It is a confusing picture. So for the moment, the best advice may come from a short French proverb: When in doubt, abstain.

In spite of all the known drawbacks, sleeping pills are used in vast quantities. It is important to understand how this can happen; otherwise you may feel that taking sleeping pills for your shift work sleep problems is "normal." You might then mistakenly feel that if you avoid or refuse to take sleeping pills you are being abnormal.

Why are sleeping pills used in such enormous quantities?

If the benefits of sleeping pills are so questionable, why is there such an enormous demand for them? Why do doctors prescribe them? And not just prescribe them now and then, but in such gigantic quantities? In 1981, 21 million prescriptions were written for sleeping pills in the United States. Here are some of the reasons why this gigantic amount of drugs was prescribed.

1. Necessity: Sleeping pills have their place. Some patients really do need, for a short time, the limited benefits that sleeping pills offer. Sometimes a patient's immediate need for sleep may be so great—for instance during critical hospitalization or after a death in the family—that the need totally outweighs the risks.

   There are also some patients, such as those suffering from depression, who need long-term use of a benzodiazepine to reduce their anxiety and help them sleep better.

2. Demand: There is an enormous demand for sleeping pills. Huge numbers of people want them and exert great pressure on doctors to supply them. A patient asking a doctor for a

sleeping pill is a little like a teenager who asks dad to borrow the family car. There is great pressure behind the request, often coupled with very small knowledge of the risks involved. Reluctantly, the doctor and dad yield to what may essentially be a reasonable request, but they issue necessary cautions and warnings. They then get similar replies: "Sure, sure. I'll be careful."

3. Cost: Visits to the doctor are costly, and the doctor knows that most patients want to avoid costly procedures. Unless a patient obviously needs to see a sleep specialist, many doctors will pick the less costly alternative for the patient and prescribe a sleeping pill.

4. Refills: Once sleeping pills have been prescribed, it can become all too easy to maintain the treatment, as Dr. E. Hartmann explains:

   "[The doctor] and the patient are likely to assume that the diagnosis was made on the first visit and that it is now merely a matter of adjusting the treatment. All that can be done is to increase the dose or change to another sleeping medication."

5. Other pressures: Besides the pressure from the individual patient on the doctor to prescribe sleeping pills, there are other important pressures. The doctor knows, for instance, that if he or she does not prescribe the pills, many other doctors will. Not the least pressure felt by the doctor comes from the pharmaceutical companies. Sleeping pills are a multimillion dollar industry, and advertisers and drug company representatives are very well equipped to present their product to doctors in the best possible light.

6. Convenience: For the staff of many institutions, it is often a lot more convenient if patients take sleeping pills so that the patients will, supposedly, have a more restful night. The staff on night shift will also be less troubled by restless patients.

Many hospitals and homes for the aged routinely give most of their patients sleeping pills every night.

7. Time factor: A doctor's time is often tightly scheduled, and patients who are sleeping poorly may not get the attention that they need. According to H. Freeman and Y. Rue:

"The persistent reply from [doctors] is still the pressure on time, the fact that these drugs are cheap [and] that they are easy to prescribe."

Do you need a sleeping pill?

A few years ago, compact cars came out with a spare tire that looked like an oversize bicycle tire. They were perfectly good for getting you to a service station but were never intended for long-term use. In fact if you kept driving your car day after day on one of these puny tires, you would be asking for trouble.

The use of sleeping pills is somewhat similar to the use of these tiny spare tires. For short-run, emergency use they can be useful, but long-term use means trouble.

For instance, if you have been kept awake night after night by anxiety, a bereavement, physical discomfort or pain, if you are in the hospital preparing for or recovering from surgery, it may make sense to take a sleeping pill for a few days. But keep in mind Dr. Hartmann's conclusion about the current use of sleeping pills: "The overall risks outweigh the overall benefits."

In contrast, the sleep "prescriptions" offered in this book involve no risks at all. There are no dangerous interactions when you use relaxation, and you can't overdose on, or become addicted to suggestion.

6

Say good-bye to those false friends of good sleep —alcohol and drugs

"You are the window through which you see the world," wrote George Bernard Shaw. "Better keep yourself nice and clean." Shaw did. He never used nicotine or alcohol, and during his ninety-four years he became England's most important playwright since Shakespeare.

Nicotine and alcohol are just two of the thousands of nonfood substances called drugs that people consume. Most of them "smudge up your windows" to some extent with their side effects. Sometimes these side effects are a reasonable price to pay if the drug will cure your sickness. But often the price is too high. This is especially the case with many drugs that we use to help us to sleep or stay awake. Nearly all of the drugs in this group bring short term gain for long-term pain.

The alcohol nightcap and why you shouldn't wear it

Alcohol taken when you are tired tends to make you get drowsy and fall asleep. This fact leads many people to use alcohol as a kind of sleeping pill, hence the expression "nightcap" for a drink taken before going to bed.

Alcohol also tends to loosen tongues; people tend to speak more freely and even to burst into song when they drink. However, lawyers, politicians, and teachers, who depend on their smooth tongues, and opera stars, who depend on their fine voices, do not normally use alcohol to improve their performance. When they do it is a sign of being "past it" or on the downhill road.

Like many sleeping pills, alcohol helps to bring unconsciousness, but this is a very different thing from healthy sleep. One of the bad features of alcohol-assisted sleep is that the important REM sleep is depressed by alcohol.

You will remember that the REM, or rapid-eyeball-motion, stage of sleep is the part of the ninety-minute sleep cycle where you almost "surface" and tend to sleep lightly and have vivid dreams for fifteen or twenty minutes. Then you plunge back down into the deep sleep of the next cycle. Sleep scientists have various theories about what the purposes of REM sleep and deep sleep may be, but they all agree that both of these stages are essential for healthy sleep. Those who use alcohol regularly as a nightcap suppress their essential REM sleep.

People who become dependent on alcohol to help them sleep often have trouble breaking this dependency. When they stop taking their alcohol nightcap, their REM sleep is no longer suppressed and rebounds, giving them wild, disturbing dreams and bad sleep. It is very often these bad dreams that drive them back to a stronger dependence on their alcohol nightcap. This can be the start of the downhill road that leads from dependence to addiction.

In spite of all of the bad effects from the alcohol nightcap, its use is widespread. At one plant, two-thirds of the shift workers used alcohol at bedtime more than once a week.

Alcohol and other drugs are enemies of good sleep. It is as dangerous to depend on them for good sleep as it is to depend on them to bring happiness.

Nicotine fits while you sleep: how to avoid them

If you are a smoker you know only too well that regularly during the day you feel the urge to light up and drag down that smoke. When the nicotine level in your body goes down, you get the urge to smoke. If you are denied a smoke when you feel like this, you experience a hunger that makes you feel agitated, a state some people call a "nic-fit."

Unless you wake up every hour during the night to have a smoke, your body will experience nicotine withdrawal all through the night, with bad effects on your sleep.

Being a smoker probably does not cause insomnia, but it certainly lowers the quality of your sleep. I well remember that one of the main benefits when I quit smoking over thirty years ago was better sleep.

What can you do about your smoking habit? Can suggestion be useful in quitting? The answer is yes, it most certainly can. After you have decided to quit, suggestion can be enormously helpful in accentuating the positive sides of quitting. But the whole process revolves around one essential. You must decide to quit. This is where the nitty gritty of quitting happens. There is an enormous difference between wanting to quit smoking and deciding to quit. People may want to quit because smoking is dangerous to their health, is a problem at work, and wastes money. So they may then go to clinics, have acupuncture, undergo hypnosis, or buy a small computer that tells them when they may smoke. Huge numbers of people do these things without having decided to quit. Without the decision it is all shoulda-coulda-woulda. The clinics and the acupuncturists take their fee, and the smoker who never made a decision to quit goes back to smoking.

So if you are a smoker who wants to quit, the one thing to concentrate on is the decision. Napoleon said that "nothing is more difficult, and therefore more valuable, than being able to make a decision." Making the decision to quit means asking yourself honestly, "Do I really want to quit?" Because, most of the time, you will do what you really want to do. If you can answer, "Yes, I really do want to quit," then you are ready to make a decision about it. From that point on, by all means take all the help you need—acupuncturists, special diets, clinics, computers.

But it is just possible that once you have made your decision to quit, you will find that you won't need any of these costly aids. Just go back to the reasons that went into your decision, pick out the positive ones, and keep suggesting them to yourself as often as you can. For example, "I sure do enjoy being able to smell this fresh air and these flowers again." Or "I sure do enjoy having all of this extra energy since I quit." And last but not least, "It's great to wake up feeling refreshed again. How much better I sleep since I quit!"

Step off the caffeine roller coaster

If you have followed the stories of Olympic athletes, you were probably impressed with how hard they train in order to become world-class challengers. Every detail counts when the difference between a gold and a bronze medal can be measured in hundredths of a second.

Shift work is similar to a challenging sports contest. To sleep well and survive shift work, you need everything going for you. Every detail counts. One of the details is the drug caffeine.

When you drink an eight-ounce mug of coffee, you take in about the same amount of caffeine as you would by drinking about three mugs of tea or a can of Coca Cola. The maximum effect is reached in thirty to sixty minutes. Since caffeine is not a food, your liver has the job of getting rid of it. After about three and a half hours your liver has reduced the amount of caffeine in your system by half.

So if you are a very heavy coffee drinker and consume two mugs every three and a half hours, your liver can't keep up with the cleanup job, and your caffeine level steadily increases. This is not good for your stomach, your health, or your sleep. It means that you are on a caffeine roller coaster, building your caffeine levels higher and higher while you are awake and then getting an uncomfortable ride when you stop drinking coffee and try to sleep.

A simple rule of thumb for caffeine is:

- Three mugs of coffee (or equivalent) max per day

- No coffee for at least four hours before sleep

That's the bad news about coffee. The good news is that caffeine is one of the few drugs that does not upset the balance of your REM and deep sleep.

If you watch these details about coffee and other drinks containing caffeine, you can enjoy both coffee and sleep.

"Uppers" that can put you six feet down

"Speed kills" was a traffic safety slogan that was adopted by drug-users many years ago. However, the "speed" that they referred to was the amphetamine/methamphetamine group of drugs, which are powerful stimulants that can have dangerous and sometimes fatal effects. These drugs appear on the street under such names as "cross-tops," "black beauties," and "pink hearts" and are used by some shift workers—especially truck drivers—to stay awake on the job.

You have seen how many powerful drugs, including alcohol, are often mistakenly used to bring sleep. Now we'll take a look at several powerful drugs that are used to prevent sleep and also at recreational drugs that are used to combat the boredom of some shift work jobs.

These drugs are not merely "false friends" and harmful to natural sleep, they can also be very dangerous. The old saying "What goes up must come down" certainly applies to these drugs. Some of the dangers lie in how rapidly and how high you will go "up"; what state you will be in while you are up there; how suddenly and, how far you will come "down"; and what state you'll be in when you get there.

Few descriptions of the dangerous effects of "uppers" and recreational drugs are more convincing and more solidly based in science than a National Transportation Board 1990 study of 182 heavy truck crashes in which the driver was killed.

This study analyzed the results of careful investigations of these accidents, which happened in a one-year period in eight states.

The key findings of this study, appearing in the report's Executive Summary, are reproduced below.

1. Of the fatally injured drivers, 33 percent tested positive for alcohol and other drugs of abuse.

2. The most prevalent drugs found were marijuana and alcohol (13 percent each), followed by cocaine (9 percent), methamphetamine/amphetamines (7 percent), other stimulants (8 percent), and codeine and phenycyclidine (PCP) (less than 1 percent each).

3. Stimulants are the most frequently identified drug class among fatally injured drivers.

4. The most frequently cited accident probable cause was fatigue (57 drivers, or 31 percent) followed by alcohol and other drug-use impairment (53 drivers, or 29 percent).

5. Of the 57 drivers who were fatigued, 19 were also impaired by alcohol and/or other drugs.

6. There is a strong association between violation of the federal hours of service regulations and drug usage.

7. There is a significant relationship between drug positive test results among professional drivers and a shipment deadline for the load being carried.

8. A disproportionately high percentage of drivers who used drugs were single, separated, or divorced.

The dangers of alcohol and drugs to drivers of all types are also shown in the table on the following page. The information in this table was obtained from several sources.

Location and sample		Alcohol only	Drugs only	Alcohol & drugs	Alcohol or drugs or both
Ontario	401 drivers killed in accidents (Warren, 1988)	43%	12%	14%	69%
U.S.	497 drivers injured in traffic accidents (Terhune, 1982)				38%
N. Carolina	600 drivers killed 1978–1981 (Owens, 1983)				14%
U.S.	440 drivers killed (Joscelyn, 1980)		51%		70%
Brownsville TN	317 tractor trailer truck drivers, one week in 1986 (Lund, 1987)				29%

Using drugs to stay awake when you are fatigued is a dangerous game. It is like getting extra credit from that very moody sleep banker. This ruthless banker can pull enough surprise demands for sleep repayment on clients who are drug-free. But to clients who use drugs to stay awake or fight boredom, the banker is often lethal. These figures prove this quite clearly.

Step 5

BANISH THE SLEEP WRECKERS

IN YOUR MIND

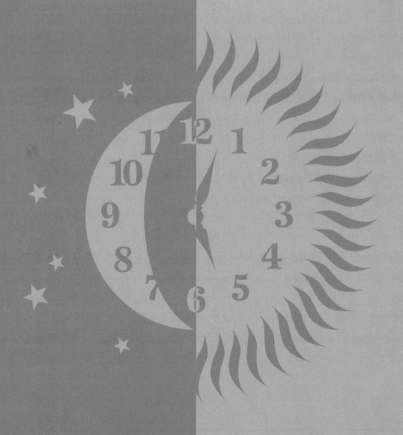

7

How to eliminate some of the worst enemies of sleep

"If my mind is at peace," a friend said recently, "I can go to sleep on a concrete floor; if it is not at peace, I will toss and turn in the most comfortable bed." My friend had put his finger on an important fact about a good night's sleep: outside disturbances and discomforts do not seem to matter nearly as much as those inside our heads.

Getting rid of these outside disturbances and discomforts is the first thing to do about your sleep troubles. So you've looked at how to change your bedroom into a sleeproom, seen the importance of a peaceful bedtime, and learned that those false friends alcohol and drugs are nearly always the enemies of a good night's sleep.

Disposing of these outside problems was the first job, but it was also the easiest job. You must now learn how to deal with all kinds of noisy troublemakers who lurk in the only place that sleep can happen—inside your own head.

How to be in control of your own mind

You want to go to sleep, but your mind is so busy it won't let you. Now if a crowd of people in your sleeproom filled it with noisy chatter, you would soon ask them to stop and be rid of them. But this noisy "chatter" is inside your own head. How do you ask it to stop? It sounds like a tough problem, dealing with these troublemakers chattering away inside your own head, but once you have pulled them out into the light where you can have a good look at them, they can be dealt with. Here is how.

The first step is to decide once and for all that you are in charge of your own mind. If you are not, then who is? "Well, nobody else is," you may answer, "but neither am I!" In that case you should turn in your driver's license. A mind that is out of control may tell its owner to drive through a red light. Driving through traffic is one of the toughest jobs that you ask your mind to handle. Obviously, you do not drive through red lights. You have decided to be in control of your mind in driving situations. In other words, when it is important for you to be in control of your mind, you control it. So if it is important for you to control your mind so that you can sleep, you will control it. That is the first very important step: to decide to be in control of your own mind.

The second step is to recognize that being in control of your own mind so that you can sleep is not always easy, but it is a skill that can be learned. What you will learn in this chapter are the skills of dealing with some powerful enemies of sleep. Their names are Worry, Regret, and Guilt. Don't underestimate them. They are heavyweights. People rarely commit suicide because their bodies trouble them. But worry, regret, and guilt cause many suicides. They also cause an enormous amount of lost sleep. Here is how to deal with them.

Worry: how to banish fear of the future

Worry is a major enemy of sleep, so let's pull this monster called worry out into the light and have a good look at him. Let's suppose you are lying in bed worrying. You would like to go to sleep but your worries about money will not let you. You've had a rush of surprise expenses lately, and now the car needs a costly overhaul. So you are worried. You just can't sleep. Your worrying goes something like this:

My bank account is overdrawn—I didn't get the raise I expected—my charge card is at its limit—there's a stack of unpaid bills—now the car needs an overhaul—but my bank account is overdrawn, etc.

Notice that this worry monster has you running in circles.

Round and round you go worrying about your problems, never getting anywhere, like a squirrel in a treadmill. Worry never comes to a conclusion. This monster knows that if you ever come to a conclusion, its power over you will end.

Worry, like most monsters, is not so terrible when you get a good look at it. Now that you know what it is doing to you, you can deal with it quite simply. Just come to a conclusion. Once you come to a conclusion about your problems, you are thinking effectively, and the worry monster slinks away.

You might come to a conclusion like this: I will talk to my bank manager about consolidating all my debts with a bank loan. Then I will update my resume and start looking for a better-paid job. Or you might even conclude that you will think about the problem tomorrow and come to a conclusion then; for now, you will sleep.

When you recognize that this terrible worry monster is just an ineffective or futile form of thinking, you can come to a very important conclusion about worry itself: you never have to worry again in your life. Never. This certainly does not mean that you never have to think again in your life, just that your thinking must be effective. So any time you catch yourself worrying, just tell yourself, "I don't have to do this." Then start thinking effectively and come to a conclusion.

This way of getting rid of worry may sound too pat and easy. That is because the worry monster is such a familiar tyrant that it seems normal for you to allow it into your life. But you don't have to be in its power if you decide not to.

What is the worst that this monster can do? What is your most frightening worry? For me, as a parent, it was that one of my children would be run over or have an accident. On a worry scale of one to ten that rated a full ten. Then one day "Buster," a friend of mine who had small children of his own, was talking about these fears. "You know, David," he said, "you just think about everything that can happen to them and do your best to protect them and warn them. Then to hell with it. Stop worrying about it. If something happens, well, you did your best to prevent it, didn't you? What more can you do?" I have never forgotten his advice. If my worst possible worry can be banished by thinking and acting effectively, I am sure not going to let silly worries about bills and charge cards keep me awake.

Regret: how to banish fear of the past

"I wish I had gotten a better education," you are saying to yourself as you try to get to sleep. "If I had only gotten that training, I would have been able to move ahead. I would have a better income, more security, and better opportunities. Only I never got the education for it."

Sound familiar? Thinking in a circle and never coming to a conclusion? Only this time the monster is called regret. The worry monster had you thinking in circles about the future; the regret monster has you running in circles thinking about the past. But you can deal with it in exactly the same way that you dealt with worry, that is, by coming to a conclusion.

For instance, in the above example you could come to conclusions like these: "I wish I had gotten a better education, but I didn't see the importance of it back then," or "I was too lazy and undisciplined at that time," or "I can start to put it right by going to night school."

We all carry a load of unfinished business from the past inside us. It may be the time, years ago, that you sold your house just before the market boomed. Or it may be the smart answer that you should have given to someone who was rude to you this afternoon. Whatever it is, the regret monster is delighted to serve this unfinished business up to you just when you want to go to sleep. Don't let it. Each time you come to a conclusion about a piece of unfinished business in your past, this monster's stock in trade shrinks.

So when it wants you to regret having sold your house just before prices took off like a rocket, come to a conclusion like this: "I did what seemed sensible at the time, but next time I will study the market more carefully." Case closed. If you are troubled about not responding to a rude comment, you might come to conclusions like these: If it is someone you know and it really bothers you, decide to bring it up with them tomorrow. If it is just a minor annoyance, resolve to be ready for them next time with a ready-to-go response like "Are you trying to be rude to me?" in case you can't think of anything better. If the rudeness came from a stranger and you couldn't think of a good reply, you may conclude that your silence was a good thing. Trading insults with strangers doesn't always pay. It's a jungle out there. Finally, as you drop the ineffective habit of thinking regretfully about the past without coming to a conclusion, the regret monster will leave you altogether.

Winston Churchill, Britain's wartime leader, usually had the gruff and menacing manner of a suspicious bulldog. He was once asked if he had any regrets about his long and active life. Churchill puffed on his cigar for a moment. "I regret betting on the red when I gambled at roulette in Monte Carlo," he answered with a twinkle in his eye.

The regret monster, no doubt, got rough handling from Churchill. You should treat it the same way.

Guilt: how to deal with this sleep wrecker

You are just about to drop off to sleep when suddenly you remember that it was your mother's birthday last week and you never even sent her a card. A hot wave of shame floods through you, banishing sleep. The regret monster has you in its power, only this time it is a special form of regret. It is one that you feel when you have offended your own value system. It is called guilt. What's to be done?

The answer is to banish the monster, again, by coming to a conclusion. If you forgot your mother's birthday, then decide to make up for it handsomely by admitting it to her and inviting her out to a special dinner. Then roll over and go to sleep.

It is natural and even healthy to feel bad when you have violated your value system. Whether this system has come to you from your parents or a religion or is one that you have assembled from many sources, it is central to what you are. If you don't respect your value system, both it and you will begin to fall apart.

Now it is one thing to feel guilt because you have violated your own value system; it is something quite different to be expected to feel guilt because you have violated someone else's value system. Some people use guilt to manipulate you and control you, often without being aware that they are doing it. "We didn't see you at our last meeting," they will say, or "You didn't send a contribution this year," or "Don't you have time for me any more?" It happens a lot. The expression "guilt trip" from the 1960s shows that people have begun to recognize manipulation by guilt. So if you find that you are being kept awake by secondhand guilt, that is, by someone's guilt trip, come to a quick conclusion about it: "Return to sender."

A final word about this powerful sleep destroyer, guilt, that the regret monster uses on you whenever it can. If you find that you have to deal with a lot of guilt in your life, consider whether one of three things is happening:

1. You have been breaking commitments, treating people badly, and generally trampling on your own reasonable value system. If so, your guilt is telling you to shape up, or risk turning into someone that you may not want to be.

2. You have been leading a life not much different from the people around you, but your very severe and demanding value system makes you feel inadequate and guilty about nearly everything.

3. You are being given a load of secondhand guilt by other people or organizations because you don't measure up to their standards.

If number 2 or 3 fits your case, it may be time to take a new look at the demands that these loads of guilt are putting on your life. Think about it carefully. Take the load of guilt off your back and have a good look at it, item by item. For each item, ask yourself, "Is there something practical that I can do about this?" If there is, then decide to do it; if there is not, put it in the trash can. You will find that there are not many items of guilt that you will want to put back on your shoulders. After all, which makes the most sense, thinking effectively, coming to a conclusion, and deciding to act on it; or letting the regret monster chase you in circles all night, jabbing you with a big stock of guilt feelings when you want to sleep?

How to calm down—and when you shouldn't

Worry, regret, and guilt tend to be chronic sleep wreckers. They can become habits. Excitement is a special-occasion sleep wrecker. Here are some examples.

You are just about to drop off to sleep on Sunday when the phone rings. Your friend wants to ask you about the exam tomorrow in the job-upgrading course you have been taking. Exam tomorrow? You thought it was on Tuesday. You had counted on having tomorrow free to do some crash studying. Now what?

Your choice is fairly clear. It is obviously better to forget about sleep and show up for the exam tired but prepared than it is to try to sleep and show up more rested, but ignorant. So if urgent planning or preparation is needed for tomorrow, forget about sleep. Plan and prepare. Rest later.

Your choice is less obvious when you are overexcited by something that does not need urgent attention. Let's suppose that you were fired today without warning. Suddenly everything in your life has changed. Paychecks will stop; the big mortgage payments on your new house will rapidly eat up your savings; your partner is looking after the kids and you cannot afford daycare. Your mind is a turmoil of rage at the unfairness of your dismissal and fear for the future. There is no urgent need to stay up all night, but in this state of mind you should not expect to sleep. Don't even try. You have taken a lot of trouble to turn your bedroom into a sleeproom, not a toss-and-turn-room. So don't go there yet. The worry monster really has you on the run this time, but by now you know what to do.

Get out a sheet of paper and a pen. Jot down a list of ideas about your former employer's actions that would support a case of wrongful dismissal. If you have some strong evidence, think about going to a lawyer. The mortgage? If worst comes to worst, you may have to sell your home. Study the house market tomorrow. Start looking for another job. Tomorrow you will prepare your resume and make a list of potential employers. A few simple plans for effective action have already tamed the worry monster and cut it down to size. You have put your problems and your conclusions on paper; they will be there in the morning. There's nothing more that you can do tonight. Now your mind is ready to listen to some suggestion about going to sleep, so turn to "The Power of Suggestion." Your sleeproom is waiting for you.

Of course not only disasters get you overexcited and rob you of sleep. Delights can keep you awake too. Suppose that this evening you and your sweetheart have decided to get married. You are excited and happy. Hundreds of thoughts crowd through your mind, making sleep impossible. So again, don't try. Make a list of all of the things that will change in your life, the actions you must take, and the arrangements that you must make. Now you have brought this happy and unruly crowd of thoughts into order by coming to some conclusions and putting it all on paper for you to deal with in the morning. You will enjoy dealing with them tomorrow, especially after a good night's sleep. Again, use suggestion as required. Sweet dreams.

Less extreme and more common than the examples above is the situation of lying in bed thinking about the car that you are going to buy or the new apartment that you are going to move into. No urgent action is needed, and there is really no conclusion to come to. Your mind is just overexcited by your intense thinking on the subject, and you can't sleep.

Former President Teddy Roosevelt had a cure for this problem. "If I can't sleep," said Teddy briskly in his usual no-nonsense manner, "I go to my desk and do some work." In this way he soon found out whether work or sleep was more important. If you have some desk work to do, you can follow Teddy Roosevelt's advice, only make sure that the work is a chore; don't reward yourself for not sleeping or it may become a habit. If you have no desk work, find some monotonous chore like tidying a cupboard, mending clothes, or cleaning the oven, and you will soon be yawning.

Switching off your job's pushy demands

Your job can take over your life. In fact, earning your living can destroy your sleep, ruin your marriage, and even threaten your life if you let it. Your job may be a jealous monster that wants you to concentrate your life on it alone. A computer used for accounting or keeping track of sales can function efficiently twenty-four hours a day. But the human brain is much more than a computer. It has the job of looking after a whole human being, and there is a great deal more to us than our jobs. A warm and loving family life, for instance, needs "love's labor," which includes love, under-standing, time, and effort.

Workaholics who give their family everything they need except themselves are very familiar types. We all know people like this, and so do the divorce courts. Besides neglecting their families, workaholics seriously neglect themselves. They do not use their time and energy outside their job to restore themselves and recreate their energies. They have no time for play. The neglected parts of a workaholic's life can be ignored and put aside during the day, but at night they clamor for attention. Workaholics often sleep badly. They have trouble getting to sleep, and their dreams are often about their work.

If your job follows you home and makes it hard for you to sleep, you may be a workaholic. People have three main reasons for becoming workaholics: (1) love, (2) fear, (3) money.

Let's look at these three reasons for workaholic behavior and learn how to deal with them.

1. Workaholics for love. It is just great if you love your work. You cannot really be a success at it unless you do. But love is one thing, obsession is another. An obsession is an unhealthy concentration on anything—a person, a drug, a job. Concentration of this kind is so demanding that the rest of a person's life is neglected and begins to wither away. Love is creative; an obsession is destructive. So if you love your work, but are neglecting your family, your friends, and yourself, your love may have become an obsession. Soon even your work will

begin to suffer from your obsession. If your sleep is already affected, your health is now in doubt. The solution is not difficult: slow down and live. If you take work home, put it aside before nine o'clock. Set aside more time for recreation. Your family relations will improve; so will your sleep.

2. Workaholics from fear—dealing with "Scrooge." Do you remember Ebeneezer Scrooge in Dickens's "Christmas Carol?" Scrooge preferred that Christmas Day be just another day at work for himself and Bob Cratchit, his clerk. If you are taking your job home with you because your boss piles more work on your desk than you can reasonably do in a day, then you may have a Scroooge-Cratchit relationship with him or her. This relationship can come in many forms. Sometimes Scrooge has a very low-key, smooth manner and may have many Cratchits working for him or her, competing fiercely for promotion, or even to hold on to their jobs. Sometimes Cratchit is an older worker trying to keep up with younger ones. But one feature is common to all of these situations: they are all based on fear. Fear of being passed over for promotion, fear of losing your job. If you suspect that you may be a Cratchit, it is time to have a talk with your boss. To start with, assume that your boss does not know about your situation. Explain things. If you find out, or if you already know, that your boss expects you always to take large amounts of work home, then you can put up with it, ask for a lighter load, or quit. If you are dreaming about your work and sleeping poorly because of overwork, your health is already being affected, so "putting up with it" means sacrificing your health to your job. Not many jobs are worth that. So, ask for a more reasonable work load, and if you do not get it, look for another job.

3. Workaholic for money. If you hold a dollar bill at arm's length, it looks like a small piece of paper with green printing on it. If you hold it right up to your nose, it fills your whole

field of vision. You can see nothing else. Some people think about money most of the time. It may be that they are always struggling to get enough money for their needs. Or it may be that they have plenty and just want more. Whatever the reason, the dollar bill is so close to their nose that they can see very little else in life. For them money has become an obsession. Their unhealthy concentration on money is destroying their life just as surely as an obsession for drugs or alcohol can. When the workaholic for money wants to go to sleep, the neglected parts of life crowd into his or her mind and cry for attention. People with obsessions rarely sleep well. If you recognize something of your own life in this description, you maybe a workaholic for money. The cure is simple. Enlarge your interests, especially your interest in other people. Take the dollar bill from in front of your eyes and hold it at arm's length where it belongs. Start to take pleasure in all of the wonderful things in life you can see now that the dollar bill is no longer in the way. Remember Ebeneezer Scrooge's office? Scrooge had nothing else left in his life, even on Christmas day, except a dollar bill on the tip of his nose.

Many other sleep-wrecking monsters wait out there besides these, but the way to deal with all of them is basically the same: drag them out into the light and have a good look at them. They all hate light. Once you can see what they are and what they are doing, they lose their power, and you can banish them. That puts you back where you belong: in charge of your own mind. Now you can suggest that it go to sleep. The next chapter shows you how to do this.

8

The power of suggestion

Say to yourself three times, "I am going to yawn."

Presto, you yawned! No drug in the pharmacy can make you yawn in three seconds, but suggestion can. This simple experiment proves that suggestion can work for you. You can therefore use suggestion to help you sleep, and this chapter will show you how.

As you saw with the yawn test, suggestion goes to work immediately. Not only that, but suggestion works better the more you use it. Few drugs in the pharmacy work better the more you use them, but suggestion does.

Not only that, but you can tailor suggestion to fit your own exact needs right now; you can write your own "suggestion sleep prescription," prepare it yourself, and take it immediately and repeatedly without fear of overdose or side effects—and all at no cost. And there is certainly no drug in the pharmacy for which all that is true.

If suggestion works so well, why isn't it widely used right now, you may ask. You'll find an answer to that as close as the nearest TV set, from which suggestions pour out in an unending stream. The whole advertising industry is largely built on the power of suggestion. Advertisers use this power to get people to do self-destructive things like smoking cigarettes or drinking alcohol, but you can most certainly learn to use it to recover a healthy natural treasure that you had as a child, namely a good night's sleep.

How does suggestion work?

We often forget that asking for something means invading someone's territory. When we ask for anything at all, we gently or not so gently shake another person's world. On the Richter scale, which measures the force with which an earthquake shakes our world, force one means a slight rattle; seven and eight on this scale means major damage. There is also a "Richter scale" in the way you use some words.

When you make a request, the scale of force goes something like this: hint—suggest—request—ask—order—demand. "Gee, Dad, my bike is too small for me now," hints the little boy a week before his birthday. A hint is an indirect and gentle way of asking. At the other end of the scale, a demand is an order from some authority that can enforce that order. "Forward march!" barks the drill sergeant as he makes a demand with the full power of the army behind him.

If a friend says to you: "I suggest that we go to the movies tonight," you do not feel under any pressure. Using the word "suggest" is the gentlest way that we can ask for something directly. The way that we use the word "suggestion" in everyday speech is a good introduction to the special way that it is used here. You will see that this gentle approach to the human mind has surprising power. It is the gentle tap on the door of the mind, which gets a friendly welcome where crude pounding fails. However, you will "hear" this gentle tap far better if you are completely relaxed. It makes perfect sense. When you relax, your guard is down. You are ready to admit friendly suggestions that knock politely at your mind's door.

How to relax your body

1. While lying on your back, clench your fists and arms as tightly as you can while you slowly breathe in. Hold your breath for a few moments. Feel the pressure in your lungs and then let it go. Relax your fists and arms as you breathe out and let go of the pressure.

2. Clench your toes and your lower leg muscles tightly while you slowly breathe in. Hold your breath for a few moments. Then

let it go. Relax your toes and lower leg muscles as you breathe out and let go of the pressure.

3. Tense up your thighs and your stomach muscles while you slowly breathe in. Hold the pressure for a few moments. Then let it go. Relax your thighs and your stomach muscles as you breathe out and let go of the pressure.

4. Tighten up your shoulders, clench your jaw, and shut your eyes tightly as you slowly breathe in. Hold the pressure for a few moments. Then let it go. Relax your shoulders, your jaw, and your eyes as your breathe out.

Now that your body is thoroughly relaxed, you are ready to quiet your mind with a creative and relaxing daydream like the one in the next section. The last section will show you how to use suggestion to go to sleep.

Use suggestion to relax your mind

Here is an example of how you can use suggestion to relax your mind:

> I am lying on a tropical beach at Cocos Cay. I am relaxing in the warm sun. I smell a pleasant hot-cotton smell from my big blue and white beach towel. The sand underneath is warm and soft and dry. I can taste the sea salt on my lips. The warm wind blows gently over my skin and I can hear the coconut palms leaves rustle overhead. The surf thunders gently on the white sand beach. Someone softly strums on a guitar. It is very peaceful. I feel wonderfully relaxed.

Let's pretend that Cocos Cay is a tropical paradise where you had the best, most relaxing holiday in your entire life. You have just used suggestion language to take yourself back there to help you relax. Let's go over this suggestion language to see how it works.

1. Imaginative. You have very skillfully used your imagination to recreate the experience of being at this peaceful place. To do this you have drawn on every sense that you have: the smell of your hot towel, the feel of the warm sun, the soft

warm sand, the wind on your skin, the taste of the salt on your lips, the sight of the blue and white beach towel, the white sand beach, the sounds of the rustling palm leaves, the gently thundering surf, and the softly strummed guitar. By appealing to all of your senses in this way you have created a vivid picture of Cocos Cay. The picture is imaginary, but the relaxation that this strongly imagined experience has brought you is quite real.

2. Personal. You have used your own personal experience in your suggestion. The strongest and richest suggestions are always based on your own experience. You can, of course, use your imagination to combine a beach from one place and a wonderful hotel from somewhere else. Or you can create an entirely imaginary experience. In each of these ways, you are using something that is personally yours.

3. Positive. Your suggested experience on Cocos Cay was entirely positive. You never mentioned that there was no screeching traffic or that the beach was unpolluted. Always make your suggestions positive. For examples, "I am feeling strong and free," not "I don't feel so weak or trapped."

4. Repetitious. The suggestion of relaxing comes at the start and also at the end of this piece. The suggestion of warmth is repeated in your vision of the sun, the towel, the sand, and the wind. The suggestion of gentleness is repeated in the sounds of the wind, the surf, and the guitar that someone is softly strumming. Repetition of these suggestions makes them much stronger. Also, if the suggestions of the whole scene of lying in the sand at Cocos Cay help you to relax, use them again. Each time that you repeat their use, the feeling of relaxation will come faster and stronger. The effect of suggestion becomes stronger with use, unlike the effects of sleeping pills.

Using suggestion to go to sleep

Sleep is like healing. If you have an injury, you must clean it up, get rid of the bacteria, and cover it up. Then leave the rest to your body. Your body is very smart. It knows how to heal an injury. Likewise, if you want to sleep, you must remove all of the things that prevent sleep. When you have done that, just leave the rest to your body. It is very smart. It knows how to sleep.

However, just as your body sometimes needs a bandage to help in the healing process, you may find that you sometimes need a suggestion bandage to help you sleep. As you saw in the last section, suggestion uses words, not chemicals, for its effects. It is now time for you to use the pharmacy that you always have with you, your rich and powerful collection of words, to help you go to sleep.

In the last section you used words freely to create a relaxing daydream; now, you just want sleep. You don't need a four course meal of words; you need a pill. Here are some simple rules to follow in making your pill in your word pharmacy:

1. Short: Your sleep prescription should be short enough to remember easily. Ten or twelve words is the maximum.

2. Simple: Concentrate on your main purpose of getting to sleep. Do not try to throw in piggyback suggestions such as dieting or quitting smoking. Do them separately some other time.

3. Reasonable: An important part of suggestion is gentleness and respect. "I must fall asleep," is an order; "I will soon fall asleep," or just the word "sleep," is a reasonable suggestion. Always make your suggestions reasonable.

4. Catchy: The words should be a carefully chosen team of words that work well together, with each word doing useful work.

5. Positive: Always make your suggestions positive. For instance, "I am feeling calm and relaxed," not "I am feeling less tense and anxious."

6. Repeated: The prescription should be repeated over and over.

7. Persistent: Remember that suggestion is the gentle knock that opens the door, but it must be a persistent gentle knock. Be patient, be persistent, and your powers of suggestion will grow stronger and stronger.

Here is an example of a sleep prescription:

Calm, tranquil, peaceful, serene
Drop, dive, plunge, fall
Sleep, slumber, doze, dream

Note that this prescription makes no false claims about how you feel now. The first line suggests calmness and then uses three more words that suggest calmness. The second line suggests the sensation of going to sleep. The very common expression "to fall asleep" is based on what we all feel like as sleep comes. Going to sleep does feel like gently falling. So use it in a suggestion and arrange the words so that "fall" and "sleep" come together. Then finally reinforce the idea of sleep with three more "sleep" words and put them in an order that sounds good: sleep slumber, doze, dream.

In these twelve words are packed the relaxed state of mind that you should be in as you go to sleep, the sensation of falling asleep, and the goal of sleep, expressed in four ways. Your suggestion sleep prescription will never be used up, it costs you nothing, you can change it or replace it any time you want without asking anyone, it can never harm you in any way, and the more that you use it the better it will work.

Before taking your prescription, say to yourself three times, "I am going to yawn." The yawn that results will focus your thinking on sleep and remind you of suggestion's power.

Let's suppose that you are going to use the prescription that I gave as an example. Say the words to yourself slowly and dreamily, letting the meaning of each word expand in your mind:

Calm, tranquil, peaceful, serene
Drop, dive, plunge, fall
Sleep, slumber, doze, dream

Then very slowly repeat the prescription. It may help to imagine a big figure "1" appearing in your mind after the first dose. You may then set this counter going so that it keeps track of how many doses of your prescription you have taken. This counter can also help to keep your mind on taking the prescription and ward off the sleep wreckers.

As sleep approaches, you may wish to shorten your prescription to the last line:

Sleep, slumber, doze, dream . . .
. . . Sweet dreams.

STEP 6

MANAGE THE SPECIAL SLEEP PROBLEMS OF SHIFT WORK

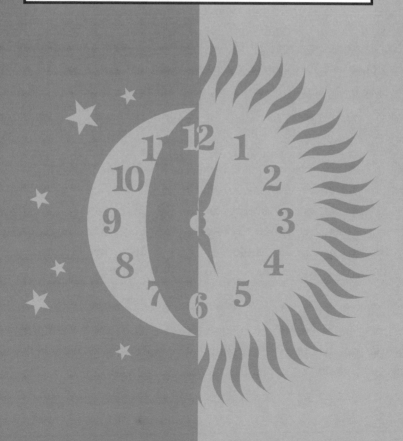

9

Sleep and shift work: your body clock meets the shift system

So far, this book has dealt with sleep problems that may affect anyone. In this chapter we look at the special sleep problems that you have as a shift worker. These problems are centered around the clash between the demands of your body clock and the demands of your shift system.

The first section deals with your body clock and will show you how to make it work for you instead of against you. The last section is on shift systems. It will show how various shift systems affect your sleep and how these systems can range from being sleep wreckers to being sleep friendly. Timetables of various systems will give you a "map" by which you can see where your own shift system fits in and how it compares with others.

Body clocks and shift systems are in this chapter together because they are both at the heart of the problem of sleep for shift workers. To solve the problem, does the shift worker have to change or does the shift system? Should the shift worker's body clocks be reset so that they fit into the shift system, or do we change the system to better fit the sleep needs of the shift worker? The answer is clear: Shift systems should be made as user-friendly as possible. Only when that has been done should the shift worker be asked and helped to adapt to the shift system.

Introducing your body clock

One of the more useful gadgets that you can buy for your home is one that automatically adjusts the temperature of your house through the day. Half an hour before you wake up in the winter it switches on the furnace so that you get up in a warm house. After you have gone to work it lowers the temperature, but raises it again just before you get home. Then it cuts back the heat again at the time you go to bed. You set it once and the rest is automatic. The purpose of this gadget, of course, is to regulate the flow of energy in your home efficiently and to avoid waste.

Your body also has a regulator or body clock, which scientists call the circadian system. It regulates the flow of your energy efficiently, turning it up to max in the morning and shutting it down at night. Besides managing the ebb and flow of energy, this clock regulates many of your body's housekeeping arrangements, including digestion, sleep cycles, and the daily rise and fall of your body temperature. In fact, sleep researchers have found that the simplest way of "reading the time" on the body clock is with a thermometer. It shows that body temperature is normally at a low point, around 98.0 degrees, at about 4:00 A.M.

On the normal setting of your body clock, your energy will peak in the morning, then there will be a dip in the afternoon (2:00–4:00 P.M.), an evening recovery, and a late evening decline, followed by the twenty-four-hour low between 2:00 A.M. and 4:00 A.M. Day shift and evening shift are clearly in tune with your body clock's regulation. It will be switching on your energy in the day when you need it and shutting it down at night when you want to sleep.

When you go on night shift, however, your body clock works against you. It will be shutting your energy down when you go on shift, and between 4:00 A.M. and 6:00 A.M. your energy and your alertness will be at their twenty-four-hour low point. Then in the morning when you come off shift and need to sleep, it will turn on your energy, so that you sleep poorly.

Your body clock can be a good friend or a tyrant, depending on how you treat it. As a shift worker, here are six important facts that you should know, starting off with just where the little rascal is to be found.

Six important facts about your body clock

1. Your body clock is located deep in your brain.

   At the point where your spinal cord joins to your brain there is a very busy network of nerves in a part of the brain about the size of a grape. This enormously important network deals with fatigue, hunger, food intake, water needs, endocrine levels, sex drive, and anger. This, one of the main crossroads of your brain, is called the hypothalamus. Within it is a tiny network of nerves called the suprachiasmatic nucleus—your body clock, or circadian system. It sits about three inches behind the bridge of your nose and is quietly giving your body instructions right now to supply the alertness you need to read this book.

2. Your body clock runs slow.

   Most people's body clocks tend to stretch the day to twenty-five hours. Research volunteers who have spent several weeks in deep caves or bunkers where daylight never shines and where there are no clocks, watches, TV, or radios, tend to get up one hour later every day. This has nothing to do with laziness; researchers can "read" the volunteer's body clock very accurately by the daily rise and fall of body temperature. Neither does this mean that nature is incapable of designing a body clock that measures days exactly; nature solves far more difficult problems. What it does mean is that for some important reason our slow body clock was a survival feature in our distant past. It can also help you survive shift work today if you keep in tune with its forward drift.

   Suppose, for instance, that after two or three weeks on an evening shift that begins at 4:00 P.M. you move to a shift that starts at midnight. Instead of going to bed at about 2:00 A.M.

after the evening shift you will now get into bed at about 10:00 A.M., eight hours later. Since your body clock is able to adjust forward an hour a day, after about a week you may have adjusted to the new shift. You are going with the flow of your body clock.

So knowledge of your slow-running body clock has a very important consequence for you as a shift worker: it tells you that if your shifts rotate from day to evening to night, following the clock, your body clock will be able to adjust to them much more easily than if they rotate backwards.

Rule: For shift rotation, clockwise is body-clock-wise.

3. Your body clock resets itself daily.

Left to itself, then, your body clock has a gentle tendency to drift forward an hour a day for its own mysterious, ancient reasons. However, since you are not living isolated in a deep cave, your body clock receives a parade of powerful time signals from all directions. Whistles blow, cocks crow, alarm clocks ring, clock radios switch on, and the smell of coffee says "wake up." All of these signals give your body clock the time and have been called "zeitgebers" (time givers) by sleep researchers ever since a German researcher first used the word.

But the most important time giver by which your body clock resets itself daily is the blazing power of the sun. This works just fine when you jet travel to a new time zone. Sunrise is the no-nonsense reminder of when the day will now begin, your body clock resets, and after a day or two of jet lag you can sleep normally. Of course your body clock is also getting many other time-giving messages in this new time zone from all the sights and sounds as people go about starting a new day. It all fits together and helps you to adjust quickly.

But when you start working night shift, your body clock gets confusing signals. While you drink your coffee and head for work, most of the world is going to bed, things are shutting down, and it is dark. No wonder it is hard to get used to night shift.

4. Melatonin can reset your body clock.

It would help if you could reset your body clock on demand. Many benefits have been claimed by the growing numbers of people who use and sell melatonin. Most of these claims, such as better sleep, delayed aging and improved sex life have yet to be proven by acceptable scientific testing. However, one very valuable property of this hormone now seems to be solidly established: melatonin can reset your body clock. In fact, melatonin is the chemical messenger or hormone that your body itself uses to tell the body clock that it is sleep time.

As the earlier section "Melatonin: magic sleeping pill?" cautioned, it is only in the last few years that there has been much research into the effects of this powerful hormone, so proceed with caution. Get your doctor's approval on your melatonin's quality and on the way that you plan to use it. Do not treat yourself like a guinea pig by experimenting with melatonin.

5. Your body clock may say that you are a "morning person" or an "evening person."

A small number of people in any group have their body clocks quite strongly set for the morning. For these "larks," morning is the best time of day. For the evening types, or "owls," however, mornings are tough, and they don't really wake up until the evening. Most people tend to be somewhere in the middle, without very big differences between their energy levels. But if mornings are easy for you, if you often wake up just before your alarm clock goes off, if you can order yourself to wake up at a certain time, if you very much dislike working at unusual times, then you are probably an extreme morning person, or lark.

Research has shown that larks have the most difficulty getting used to night shift, even if they work night shifts all the time. If this sounds like you, if you are an extreme lark, then maybe your chances of ever getting used to night shift are poor, and night shifts are not for you.

6. Your body clock, like all clocks, is delicate.

Your body clock is a delicate instrument and should be treated with respect. To yank it off night shifts just when it is getting used to them and then to ask it to adjust to nights again just when it has recovered, is asking for trouble—sleep trouble. You should either let it adjust to a long stretch of night shifts or else hustle through the night shifts so quickly that it doesn't adjust at all. Anything in between spells trouble.

Rule: More than twenty-one or less than three night shifts in a row are easy on your body clock; they give it a chance to adapt properly or not at all.

The next section will show you how well various shift systems treat your body clock and your sleep needs.

Shift systems and sleep: how to rate them

"You lift a large sack of coal to your shoulders," a steel worker wrote in the year 1919, "run towards the white hot steel in a 100-ton ladle, must get close enough without burning your face off to hurl the sack, using every ounce of strength, into the ladle and run, as flames leap to roof and the heat blasts everything to the roof. Then you rush out to the ladle and madly shovel manganese into it, as hot a job as can be imagined."

The steelworker who described these working conditions for the Interchurch World Movement worked an average eighty-four-hour week in a four-week cycle. This cycle, half twelve-hour day shifts and half twelve-hour night shifts, included one crossover shift of twenty-four hours. This incredibly harsh shift system was not uncommon among steelworkers in 1912. At that time almost half of them worked over seventy-two hours per week, and almost one quarter worked eighty-four or more hours per week. The effects of such a system on the health, sleep needs, family life, and social life of the shift worker can only be imagined. For instance, the steelworker who described his work at the furnaces went on to describe his routine when coming off night shift:

6:00 A.M. Leave work after 12 hour night shift

6:45 A.M. Bathed, breakfast

7:45 A.M. Asleep

4:00 P.M. Wake up, put on dirty clothes, eat supper, get pack of lunch

5:30 P.M. Report for work

Since this is about the worst possible shift system, it is a useful starting point. You can use it as a zero to rate other shift systems by, including your own. The chart below shows how this steelworker's schedule looks in a timetable. "D" or "N" means 12 hour day or night shifts; "d," "e," or "n" means 8-hour shifts; "–" means day off.

Steelworker's shifts—1919

	M	T	W	T	F	S	S	
Week 1	D	D	D	D	D	D	D	1. Shifts: 12 hours
Week 2	D	D	D	D	D	D	D/N	2. Shifts rotate: After 2 weeks
Week 3	N	N	N	N	N	N	N	3. Rotation: Head to tail
Week 4	N	N	N	N	N	N	–	4. Hours/week work: 84 average!
								5. Days off/week: 1/4
								6. Weekends off: None!
								7. Total time off/wk: 84 hours!

A schedule like this is fine if you are a robot made out of steel and transistors, but not if you are a human being. Where is the time for playing with the kids, visiting friends, or going to a meeting? Normal time for these activities is from 6P.M. to 10P.M. on weekdays and from 9:00 A.M. Saturday or Sunday morning to midnight. This works out to twenty hours of social time on weekdays, and thirty hours on weekends for a total of fifty hours per week. Here is how the steelworker's social time schedule looks:

Steelworker's social time off—1919

	M	T	W	T	F	S	S	Totals
Week 1	2	2	2	2	2	2	2	14
Week 2	2	2	2	2	2	2	0	12
Week 3	0	0	0	0	0	0	0	0
Week 4	0	0	0	0	0	0	6	6

32 hours, or 8 hours/week average

What a grim schedule. Instead of the fifty hours/week of social time that a day shift worker gets now, the steelworker got only fourteen on his best week, and no weekends off at all, ever.

How about sleep? Quality time for healthy sleep is 10:00 P.M. to 6:00 A.M., making a total of fifty-six hours per week. Let's see how much of this quality sleep time the poor steelworker got:

Steelworker's quality sleep time—1919

	M	T	W	T	F	S	S	Totals
Week 1	6	6	6	6	6	6	6	42
Week 2	6	6	6	6	6	6	0	36
Week 3	0	0	0	0	0	0	0	0
Week 4	0	0	0	0	0	0	6	6

84 hours, or 21 hours/week average

A tough sleep schedule. Instead of averaging fifty-six hours of prime sleep time per week, the steelworker averages only twenty-one hours.

Let's follow the steelworker at the end of his day shift. He leaves work at 6:00 P.M., has two hours for travel, cleanup, and a meal and then has two hours of social time before going to bed at 10:00 P.M. However, since he has to be at work at 6:00 A.M., he has to get up at 4:00 A.M. and so gets only six hours of sleep. To get eight hours he would have to go to bed after finishing dinner at 8:00 P.M., which means no time for family or friends.

Thanks to labor's long and sometimes bloody struggles, such shift work is a thing of the past in the U.S. and other advanced countries. Now let's look at some of today's shift systems.

Common shift system in U.S.

The most common rotating shift system in the U.S. today is the one shown below. It is an enormous improvement on the steelworker's shift, but it is also an out-of-date system. Even if you are not working this system, look at the diagram and you will quickly spot its drawbacks: rapid anticlockwise rotation makes it hard to adapt to the new shift, and by the time you do, the shifts change. There is only one weekend off in four, and few days off. This system is needlessly hard on workers, on their families, and on productivity too. It is time for it to join the 1919 Steelworker's system in a museum.

Common shift system in U.S. today

	M	T	W	T	F	S	S	
Week 1	d	d	d	d	d	–	–	1. Shifts: 8 hours
Week 2	–	–	n	n	n	n	n	2. Shifts rotate: After 7 days
Week 3	n	n	–	–	e	e	e	3. Rotation: Counterclockwise (harmful)
Week 4	e	e	e	e	–	e	e	4. Hours/week work: 42 average!
								5. Days off/week: 1.75 week
								6. Weekends off: 1 in 4, or 25%
								7. Hours/week off: 126

Here is how the social time schedule looks for this very common shift system.

Common shift system: social time off

	M	T	W	T	F	S	S	Totals
Week 1	4	4	4	4	4	15	15	50
Week 2	4	4	4	4	4	4	4	28
Week 3	4	4	4	4	0	0	0	16
Week 4	0	0	0	0	4	4	4	12
								106 hours or 27 hours/week average

Social time off for Week 1, which is a normal day shift worker's week with the weekend off, is at the fifty hours maximum. After that week, social time nose dives, and in the last two weeks is starting to look as bad as the 1919 steelworker's weekly totals.

Common shift system: social time off

	M	T	W	T	F	S	S	Totals
Week 1	8	8	8	8	8	8	8	56
Week 2	8	0	0	0	0	0	0	8
Week 3	0	8	8	8	4	4	4	36
Week 4	4	4	4	4	8	8	8	40

140 hours or 35 hours/week average

Quality sleep time also starts at maximum in Week 1 with fifty-six hours. Then it drops way down with the night shifts in Week 2. Then it picks up in the last two weeks. Added to the rapid counter-clockwise shift rotation, this irregular pattern of quality sleep hours is needlessly hard on the shift worker. The popular "compressed week" shift systems looked at below offer some attractive modern alternatives.

Compressed week shift systems

The increasingly popular "compressed week" system features four twelve-hour shifts (two days, two nights) followed by four days off, and is often known as the "platoon" or "firefighter's" shift system. The basic system has two twelve-hour days, two twelve-hour nights and four days off: (DDNN- - - -). There are several variations of this, such as (DDDD- - - -NNNN- - - -) and even (DDNN- - - - -). These twelve-hour shift systems are now common for firefighters and chemical and petroleum workers and have also been successfully introduced widely, including in the mini-steel industry.

An advantage of the two days followed by two nights version of this system is that your body clock doesn't even begin to adapt to night shifts by the time they are over. Reducing the number of night shifts in a cycle goes even further with the four-on-and-five-off (DDNN- - - - -) system, largely adopted by nurses in British Columbia in 1993. It has only two night shifts in a nine-day cycle.

Here is the common form of the platoon or firefighter's system.

Compressed week shift system (platoon system)

	M	T	W	T	F	S	S	
Week 1	D	D	N	N	–	–	–	1. Shifts:12 hours
Week 2	–	D	D	N	N	–	–	2. Shifts rotate: After 2 days
Week 3	–	–	D	D	N	N	–	3. Rotation: Clockwise
Week 4	–	–	–	D	D	N	N	4. Hours/week work: 42 average
Week 5	–	–	–	–	D	D	N	5. Days off/week: 3.5 week
Week 6	N	–	–	–	–	D	D	6. Weekends off: 3 in 8, or 37.5%
Week 7	N	N	–	–	–	–	D	7. Hours/week off: 126
Week 8	D	N	N	–	–	–	–	

Social time off in this system is compressed into the abundant days off; on day and night shifts it is the same as the steelworker had.

Compressed week: social time off

	M	T	W	T	F	S	S	Totals
Week 1	2	2	0	0	4	15	15	38
Week 2	4	2	2	0	0	15	15	38
Week 3	4	4	2	2	0	0	15	27
Week 4	4	4	4	2	2	0	0	16
Week 5	4	4	4	4	2	2	0	20
Week 6	0	4	4	4	4	2	2	20
Week 7	0	0	4	4	4	15	2	29
Week 8	2	0	0	4	4	15	15	40

228 hours, or 29 hours/week average

The weekly totals of social time off in the compressed week vary much less than in the common shift system. Although the weekly average of social time is only two hours more than it is for the common shift system, the big four-day-off time blocks, and the greater number of weekends off (38 % compared to 25 %) make this system very popular.

Compressed week: quality sleep time

	M	T	W	T	F	S	S	Totals
Week 1	6	6	0	0	6	8	8	34
Week 2	6	6	6	0	0	8	8	34
Week 3	8	6	6	6	0	0	8	34
Week 4	8	8	6	6	6	0	0	34
Week 5	8	8	8	6	6	6	0	42
Week 6	0	8	8	8	6	6	0	36
Week 7	0	0	8	8	8	6	6	36
Week 8	6	0	0	8	8	8	6	36

282 hours or 35 hours/week average

The quality sleep time during this eight-week cycle varies very little from the thirty-five hour average. Combined with the short two-day night shift, which is over before you adapt to it, this shift system has far healthier sleep conditions than the common shift system. Also, its more generous recreation time and weekends off make for more chances for relaxation.

However, it is important to remember that on the days when you have a twelve-hour shift you are back in 1919 with the steelworker. There is really no time for anything except eating, sleeping, travel, and work. But unlike the steelworker, you can look forward to those four days off.

A huge variety of rotating shifts exist besides the ones shown here. When you put them on timetables in this way, it makes it much easier to compare them and spot their good and bad features.

Fixed shift systems

If you are a nurse or a police officer, the chances are that you are working a fixed shift. These fixed, or nonrotating, shift systems are common in the U.S., especially in these occupations. Usually, the senior or more highly qualified staff work the popular day shifts and the junior members get the evening or night shifts. The main advantage of this system is that if you are on evening or night shift you are able to settle down, adapt to it, and sleep better than you would on a rotating shift system. Also, many workers prefer shift evening or night work to day work, especially those who like to avoid crowds or prefer less supervision in their work.

However, if you are on fixed night shifts and are finding it impossible to get used to this schedule, you may be a morning type. As described in the last section, a small minority of people have body clocks strongly set for maximum alertness in the mornings. This group does not adapt to night shift.

In general, day shifts are the most popular, and most workers on fixed shifts are eager to move to days. This system therefore encourages workers to switch jobs rarely and to build up seniority to get the desirable day shifts.

Irregular shift systems

Many U.S. workers are on irregular shifts, mostly workers in transportation such as truck drivers, bus drivers, and train and airline crews. These systems can be very hard on the shift worker, especially as regards to sleep quality, unless there is enough built-in time off to smooth out the bumps. If you want to compare your irregular shift system with the other ones here, you will need to keep track of them over ten or even twenty weeks to get a fair sample.

How to rate your own shift system

How does your shift system, or the one that you are being offered, rate? You may get some good (or bad) surprises when you fill in the blanks below and compare your system closely with these systems, ranging from the ancient steelworker's system to the modern platoon system.

My shift system at _____

```
         M  T  W  T  F  S  S
Week 1                              1. Shift length:_____hours
Week 2                              2. Shifts rotate: After _____days
Week 3                              3. Rotation: clock/counterclock
Week 4                              4. Hours/week work:___average
Week 5                              5. Hours/week nights:___average
Week 6                              6. Days off:____/week
Week 7                              7. Weekends off: ___in___or___%
Week 8                              8. Hours/week off:____hours
```

My shift system: social time off

Remember that social time is from 6:00P.M to 10:00P.M. weekdays and from 9:00 A.M. to 12:00 midnight Saturday and Sunday. This adds up to twenty hours for the weekdays and thirty hours for the weekend, making a total of fifty hours maximum per week. Allow time before a shift starts and after it ends for preparation, cleanup, and travel.

```
         M  T  W  T  F  S  S       Totals
Week 1
Week 2
Week 3
Week 4
Week 5
Week 6
Week 7
Week 8
```

My shift system: quality sleep time

The best hours for quality sleep are from 10:00 P.M. to 6:00 A.M. The more of this time that your shift system allows, the better. Make the same two-hour allowance before and after shifts for travel, as above.

```
         M  T  W  T  F  S  S       Totals
Week 1
Week 2
Week 3
Week 4
Week 5
Week 6
Week 7
Week 8
```

Now that you have the numbers together for your shift system, you can enter them in the table below and compare them with the three other shift systems ("Worst," "Typical" and "Compressed")

Table to compare your shift system with others

	Worst 1919 Steelworker	Typical 1994 Common	Compressed "Platoon" "Firemen"	Your System (fill in)
Number of shifts	2	3	2	_____
Number of crews	2	4	4	_____
Shifts rotate every	14 days	7 days	8 days	_____
Rotate	clockwise	no	yes	_____
Night shifts in a row	14	7	2	_____
Hours work/week	84 hrs	42 hrs	42 hrs	_____
Days off/week	0.25	1.75	3.5	_____
Weekends off	0	1/4 (25%)	3/8 (38%)	_____
Total time off/week	84 hrs	126 hrs	126 hrs	_____
Social time off/week	14 hrs	37 hrs	48 hrs	_____
Quality sleep time/week	21 hrs	35 hrs	35 hrs	_____

The time of your life: how much do you sell?

How does overtime affect your shift system and your sleep system? At what stage does overtime become overwork?

Many workers are glad to get overtime. Raising a family and just paying for necessities these days takes a lot of cash. Since 1972, the real income of most blue-collar Americans has declined. That means that a paycheck for the same hours on the same job today pays fewer bills than it did back then. Overtime helps to make up the difference. Also, with the decline in job security, it makes sense to "make hay while the sun shines." Those secure, jobs-for-life are a thing of the past, and a nest egg can be essential in case your company starts to do some downsizing. So, "the more overtime the merrier!" many workers are saying.

Overtime has certainly grown merrily in recent years. From 1970 to 1985, the average overtime for U.S. workers in manufacturing ranged from 2.5 to 4.0 hours per week. Now it is around 5.0 hours per week. Part of the increase is due to the economic recovery, but according to the *Wall Street Journal*, the change may be long lasting:

"The cost of health insurance and other benefits for new workers has made paying overtime to current employees a bargain . . . (because) blue-collar benefits now average $5.62/hour . . . So it's cheaper to pay overtime to a $10-per-hour worker (at time-and-a-half that costs $15 an hour) than to hire a worker at the same base wage plus benefits ($15.62 an hour). And by paying overtime, the employer avoids the cost of training a new worker."

According to this article some of the increases have been too much of a good thing. General Motors workers went on strike at the Flint, Michigan, plant because they were required to work overtime that resulted in sixty-six hour weeks.

Steelworkers at Allegheny Ludlum struck in the spring of 1994 after being forced to work as much as 146 hours in two weeks. That works out to seventy-three hours per week. One worker at Allegheny had to work forty-two days without a day off last year. The pressure on workers to work overtime is widespread. The U.S. Department of Labor reports that overtime is at its highest level since they began keeping track in 1956. Many employers now discipline or fire workers who refuse overtime. The bad effects of forced overtime on your family life, your health, and your sleep are not hard to see.

If you gladly work overtime to help pay your bills, that's fine, but being forced to work overtime repeatedly against your will is something very different. It boils down to an attempt by employers to return to the labor practices of the past. What can you do about it?

Not much unless you belong to a union, and even unionized workers have had to go on strike to try to prevent forced overtime. Without a union, you have no clout at all, and 83 percent of the U.S. workforce is nonunion. The United States has fewer unionized workers today than any other advanced industrialized country in the world. Since the 1980s U.S. industry has moved from the "Rust Belt" of the northeast to the "Sun Belt" of the southwest, a move from a union-strong to a union-weak area. The decent working conditions and good wages that most American workers have enjoyed did not come without a struggle. It was fought by workers who had clout because they were organized in unions. Nonunion workers have enjoyed the benefits of these struggles too, and in a way have had a free ride. Unless workers bargain collectively through their union, the free ride will be over, and the hard-won benefits will be lost. Among them will be the right to refuse overtime when you don't want it.

Workers who are eager for more overtime should learn from this story of a Russian peasant:

"You can have as much land," the big landowner told this Russian peasant long ago, "as you can circle on foot before sunset today." The excited peasant set out at a run to encircle a huge block of land, but as sunset approached he had still not closed his circuit. Running as hard as he could, staggering and falling, the peasant collapsed and died of exhaustion without reaching his goal. In this story by Leo Tolstoi, titled "How Much Land Does a Man Need?" the great Russian writer offered a grim answer to this question: Just about six feet is all we need eventually, and we will get it soon enough without an assist from overwork.

Making arrangements for people to work themselves to death was possible in old Russia, but not in modern America. However, without the clout of a union behind them, workers on their own may easily today face the choice of overworking themselves into ill-health or refusing and being fired.

Getting a better shift system: examples

Bad habits are often hard to break. Everyone knows smokers who can't seem to quit. In spite of the inconvenience, the cost, and the grim medical evidence they keep lighting up. It is often the same with a bad shift system. The shift workers can tell you in great detail what is wrong with it. The company can't really remember just where the shift system came from, and they know that it isn't perfect, but they stick with it. "If it isn't broke, why fix it?" they will say, or "Why rock the boat?"

In this section you will meet managements that were not afraid to "rock their boats" and make changes to their shift systems. These changes made big improvements to worker job satisfaction, to productivity, and in one case, to the bottom line of the company's income account.

Case #1—Great Salt Lake Minerals & Chemicals Corporation: About forty miles north of Salt Lake City on the east side of the Great Salt Lake, miners operate front-end loaders to scoop up potash from evaporation ponds. This mining operation ran on a normal three-shift system with weekly shift changes. The shifts rotated so that after a week on night shift (midnight to 8:00 A.M.) you would move to evening shift (4:00P.M. to midnight), and after a week on that shift you would move to day shift (8:00 A.M. to 4:00 P.M.). This system, which rotates to the previous shift, is called a counterclockwise system. The mine had operated on this weekly counterclockwise shift rotation system for ten years.

Many workers were unhappy with this shift system. A complaint made by 81 percent of the shift workers was that this weekly shift change was too rapid and that it took from two to four days or more to adjust to the new sleep schedule following shift changes. Some workers (26 percent) could never adjust before being rotated again. Efficiency was obviously affected, as 29 percent reported falling asleep at work at least once in the previous three months.

In 1980 the company wisely allowed a team of sleep researchers to experiment with an improved shift system. This system was designed to be in harmony with the worker's body clocks, which can adjust much more quickly to clockwise shift changes than to counterclockwise changes. The new system reversed the direction of shift rotation to clockwise and split the shift workers into two groups. One group was on a weekly shift rotation; the other was on a three-week rotation.

The results of these changes were analyzed after nine months of operation; they were remarkable. The production of potash increased by about 10 percent, worker turnover dropped from 50 percent to

30 percent, and worker sleep quality, health, and satisfaction with the system all improved.

Shift workers' first choice was the three-week, clockwise rotating shift system. The clockwise shift change made it much easier for workers' body clocks to adapt to a new shift, and the three-week period gave them a chance to settle into a system and get used to it. Such changes to modern shift systems are becoming more common.

Case #2—The Philadelphia Police Department: In 1986 the department was on an old-fashioned eight-day counterclockwise rotating shift system. It did not work well. Sleep problems were reported by 50 percent of the officers, and the rate of accidents on night shift was four times the day rate. After changing to an eighteen-day clockwise system, they experienced a 25 to 30 percent decline in sleeping on the job, a 40 percent drop in accidents, and a five times increase in family satisfaction with the new system.

How you can get a better shift system

If you are sleeping badly due to a bad shift system, you can do three things:

1. You can grumble and put up with it;

2. You can get mad and quit; or

3. You can take some well-chosen steps to change the system.

This section will help you plan those well-chosen steps. So let's imagine that you suspect your sleep problems are due to a bad shift system. Being a loyal employee, you want to try to change the system in a spirit of cooperation and goodwill. You know that this will not be easy. As K. Kogi wrote in *Introduction to the Problems of Shiftwork*: "Although most current shift systems could be greatly improved, there is considerable inertia and a tendency to stick to the ongoing system . . . changing it requires considerable effort."

Nevertheless, you firmly believe that not only will you and your fellow workers benefit from the change, but your employer will too. You are after a "win-win" change.

Change takes power, and as an individual you have little power. But "knowledge is power." This leads to the first of the three steps you should take:

1. Do your homework: Obtain knowledge, inform yourself. Find out the answers to these questions:

   ■ Where did the present shift system come from? Has it been thoroughly overhauled within the last five years? If so, your chances of changing it are not good. A change of shift system is an upset that most organizations, especially large ones, don't want too often. If it has just been cobbled and patched together from time to time over the years, that's different; a complete change may be just what it needs.

   ■ What is wrong with the present system? Do the shifts rotate clockwise? How many night shifts are there in a row? How about weekends off and social time off per week? This is where making a timetable of your system and rating it as shown in the last section can be a big help. It will give you the facts and figures you need to convince others.

   ■ Do your fellow workers complain about sleep problems, rapid shift rotation, and lack of social time off?

   ■ How about the other telltale signs of a bad system: absenteeism, low morale, sickness, accidents and injuries, a high staff turnover rate, low productivity, defective production or service, and equipment breakdowns?

   ■ Are there other businesses or organizations similar to yours that have different shift systems? Are their workers content with their system? How successful are these operations?

   ■ How about the new system you would like to see brought in? When you compare its features in a table with your present system, is it a clear winner? If there are several possible new systems to choose from, put them all in your table to see how they stack up. A shift system change has a big effect on people's lives; your homework must show that it will be a good effect.

2. Try out your ideas: Now its time to try out your ideas on your fellow shift workers. You have done your homework and are well prepared to show the good reasons for a change. But don't be discouraged if you run into some opposition. People get used to a system, and change takes effort. A bad shift system can be just like a bad habit: hard to break. Someone is bound to say, "If it's not broken, why fix it?" Try asking them if that is the way they run their car. Or ask them if they would like to fly with an airline that used that saying as a slogan. The point you are making, of course, is that a smart person fixes things before they break.

3. Present your ideas: You have been patiently explaining your ideas to your fellow shift workers, and you have also carefully listened to their ideas. Your plan for a change to the shift system is one that most of them now support. It is time to present your ideas. This takes tact. What you will be doing, in effect, is reaching over from the back seat and tapping the driver on the shoulder. As well as tact, it also calls for a change of tactic. You are now trying to convince management that a new shift system will improve productivity as well as increasing workers' job satisfaction. You can point to the example of the Salt Lake potash mining operation mentioned in the last section. The idea of improving a business's bottom line is a powerful argument.

In a large operation that is unionized, you should approach your union representative. Some large operations that are not unionized have worker-management committees to improve efficiency. If so, try presenting your ideas to them. In large businesses that have no structured way for workers to present ideas to management and that are not worker-friendly, tread with care. Any kind of organizing for change by workers may be seen as a threat.

In smaller businesses that are not unionized, try approaching a sympathetic junior manager. If he or she likes your ideas for a better shift system and wants to pick up the ball and run with it, that's great. Let that person take the credit; your reward is a better shift system and a good night's sleep.

10

Evening shifts:
four ways to survive them
and sleep well

◆

"Night shift kills the body; evening shift kills the family" goes a grim proverb.

As with many proverbs, this one holds a lot of truth. The problems of night shift can kill you. They can kill you quickly if you fall asleep on the job or driving home. They can also kill you slowly. The stress of night shift from long-term poor sleep and bad diet can shorten your life; many research studies and figures back this up.

The problems of evening shift can "kill" your family. Evening shifts wipe out the valuable social hours from 6:00 P.M. to 10:00 P.M. when most family time together during the week happens. For their families, shift workers on steady evening shifts are like ghosts who make noises late at night and are never around in daytime. For evening shift workers, their families, too, seem like ghosts; they are around somewhere at night, but they vanish with daylight.

However, once you know that evening shifts are a threat to your family and your social life you can arm yourself against these dangers. This chapter and the next will help you to survive the hauntings of evening and night shift so that your sleep, your health, and your family are all protected. The bad effects of these shifts can be avoided. Here are four ways to help you survive evening shifts.

Sleep strategies

At first glance, your sleep when you work evening shift does not seem to be a problem. Although you may not get into bed until 1:00 or 1:30 A.M., most of your sleep will be in normal hours when your neighborhood is at its darkest and quietest. Also, you can sleep in as late as you want. You should have no trouble logging eight hours before your body clock begins to turn on your morning energy surge after 9:00 A.M. If you live alone and if your social life fits in with daytime hours, evening shift has no sleep problems for you.

But if you live with your family, and especially if you are a single parent, you will at least be disturbed by the family getting up, and you may even have to get up yourself at 6:00 or 7:00 A.M. to put breakfast on the table. This means that you have had five hours sleep at most, which is not enough. Here are three ways to get your full eight hours.

First, the ideal way is to have a spouse or baby-sitter handle breakfast for the family while you sleep in. Second, you can duck back into bed as soon as everyone has left and try to make up your eight hours before 11:00 A.M. The trouble with this plan is that while you are trying to get back to sleep, your body clock is starting to turn your energy on. If this still leaves you short of rest, you can try the third option, which is to sleep in the early afternoon before leaving for your shift. The advantage of sleeping at this time is that it fits in with your midafternoon energy dip and goes with your body clock's regulation instead of trying to fight it.

Whatever way works for you, stick with it—make it a regular routine and give your body a chance to get used to it. This means that on days off, too, you should try not to stray too far from your workdays' sleep schedule.

Another important concern about your daytime sleep is to protect it from "nibblers." Nibblers are people who know that you work shifts but think it's OK to ask you to do little jobs during the day, to go out and do some shopping, or answer the phone. Kindly and firmly let them know that you need your sleep just as they need theirs.

Above all, get enough sleep. Studies show that shift workers on evening shift have a daily average of only 6.5 hours sleep. So keep on good terms with your sleep "banker." Keep track of how many hours sleep you get each night and write it down. Don't build up a sleep debt.

Protect your family life

If you are a family man or woman, going on evening shift means leaving in time to be at work at 3:00 or 4:00 P.M. This means that when your children and spouse are home from school or work, you are at work, and by the time the shift is over the kids are in bed. While you are on evening shifts you may rarely see your kids. Protecting your bond with them needs special efforts. Here is what to do.

First, before you start evening shifts, have a family meeting and explain to the kids what evening shift work is and how long you expect to be on it. Let them know that you will miss seeing them, but that you will try to make the time with them quality time. Ask them if they can think of ways to keep in touch better. It may all sound very obvious, but children like to know exactly what is going on and where they fit in. It will make them happy just to know that you are concerned about them. It's a good idea to have a big calendar or bulletin board where they can see when you have shifts and when the days-off treats and outings will happen. Children's time sense is undeveloped. Next week might as well be next year for them. Marking the days off on a calendar helps them to deal with time and learn about it.

Second, you can keep in touch with notes and letters. Kids love them. Also, ask them to leave their schoolwork out for you to look at, and then write encouraging comments. Children thrive on praise. Once in a while you can do a Santa Claus number and leave some goodies by their bedsides. But the main thing they miss is you, so struggle out at breakfast from time to time. Avoid the heavy parent scene at these breakfasts ("What's all this I hear . . . ?"). Make them happy occasions.

Third, make plans to give your children quality time on your days off. It's a good idea to include them in the planning to avoid disappointments. You can do this by writing them notes or talking it over at one of your breakfast appearances. When the day off comes, don't appear crabby or groggy. Invest plenty of hours in sleep while you are on those evening shifts, and enjoy your days off by being well rested. Keep your sleep bank account full with regular eight-hour deposits.

Finally, if you find that you are stuck on steady evening shifts and your family life is suffering, try to trade with someone who is on night shift. If all else fails, update your resume and go job hunting. One advantage of evening shifts is that you can easily schedule job hunting and interviews. Any job that threatens your family should be considered temporary.

Keep your social life alive

If evening shifts make it hard to keep in touch with your family, what chance do your friends have? Evening shifts cut right across those prime social hours in the evening. Barbecues, dinners, parties, bowling, dances, sporting events, clubs, and societies are all going full blast while you are on evening shift. It is bad enough missing out on all these good times, but you're also suffering a less obvious loss. When your friends plan these events and wonder who to ask, they may rate you as a probable no-show because of shift work, and scratch your name from their list. The same thing can happen in clubs and societies. Shift work makes it impossible to guarantee that you will be able to function fully as a member of organizations. Over the months, your evening shifts can quietly strangle your social life. The more you realize that this is happening, the less well you will sleep. Here is what to do to prevent it.

First, make a timetable of your shifts for the next month or two and pass out copies to everyone you want to keep in touch with. Hand them out, mail them, fax them. Get them out there. Your spouse can help. This does two things: it lets your social contacts know exactly when you are free, and it lets them know that you care about keeping in touch with them.

Second, keep in touch in other ways. Phone friends at work during the day, arrange a blitz of get-togethers on your days off. Some clubs or societies may be glad for your help during daytime hours—give it to them. Make an effort; struggle against the strangling of your social life.

Lastly, one of your most important social contacts is a buddy, a pal—a fellow shift worker who knows the crazy world of shift work from the inside. Someone who will always listen to your troubles, just as you will listen to his or hers. This person may be your most important social contact of all. Look after this friend.

Making these efforts to help your social life survive will bring many benefits, among them more peace of mind and better sleep.

How to have evening shift security

Since you are normally awake until 10:00 P.M. or midnight, the danger of dozing off during evening shift is not usually a problem. The safety and security concerns on this shift come not from yourself, but from others.

If you are a woman working evening shift, you have two main safety and security concerns. First, while you are on the job you may be threatened by other workers or by the public. Second, when you leave your workplace sometime after midnight, you may be threatened in parking areas, on the streets, or while using public transit, by men who saw you at your workplace or who meet you by chance. Some workplaces are located in areas where a man doesn't feel safe alone at night, either. The best way to deal with these problems is by getting together with other employees and taking group action. Explain any problems to management or your union. A buddy system, carpooling, security guard escorts, or relatives or friends who can pick you up and see you safely home will end your anxieties.

If you are a man with a wife and family at home, or a single parent with children at home (even with a baby-sitter) while you are on evening shift, you may sometimes be anxious about their safety. If all of your friends and relations know that they should phone before visiting, family members need not answer the door to any unexpected callers while you are at work. When they answer the phone, they can just say that you are unavailable and ask the caller to leave a number.

A good way to feel closer to your family is to wear a pager, or even carry a cellular phone, so family member can reach you quickly. Routine check-in calls at set times can give all of you security and peace of mind.

Finally, beware of falling asleep while driving home. Don't nod off and perish; pull over, take a ten-minute nap, and survive.

11

Night shifts: five ways
to survive them and sleep well

The sleep problems of night shift are the heart of this book. As you read the first chapters, you began preparing for better sleep. Now it is time for you to become a sleep champion. A rodeo champion was once asked the secret of his success. "Before I go in the corral," he answered, "I imagine a perfect ride. Then I just go in and do it." Being a champion means having a very clear idea of the steps that you are going to take. Here are five steps to put you in the champion class of shiftwork sleepers.

How to get a good day's sleep

You are just getting home after a long night shift. You congratulate yourself again on having chosen a quiet part of the city to live in. Just before you open your front door you nod to your neighbors. That friendly visit you made when you gave them your shift timetable will pay off again today. They will put off using noisy appliances like saws and lawn mowers until the afternoon.

A hot shower helps you to relax and while you eat a light breakfast, you watch a soothing National Geographic TV special on coral reefs. If any thoughts of work come into your mind, you gently push them out. You avoid bringing the job home with you—unless you have had a troublesome shift and need to phone a fellow shift worker and talk it out.

Back in the bathroom to clean your teeth, you notice some sleeping pills in the cupboard. You haven't used one of those for about six months. You reach for the bottle, take the lid off, and dump them all in the toilet. Good riddance. This reminds you of two more drugs that you have said good-bye to: the alcohol nightcap that used to knock you out for a while but then gave you rotten sleep and the cigarettes that helped ruin the quality of your sleep and gave you coughing fits when you woke up. Good riddance to them too.

You relax in front of the TV and watch the tropical fish for a few minutes. You yawn and switch off the set. You put the phone answering machine on the one-ring-and-take-a-message setting and turn down the volume. Now it's bedtime.

Some of your friends on night shift don't go to bed when they get home. They stay up all morning during their morning energy surge and then go to bed at midday. You prefer to get into bed as soon as possible after the shift is over. You have tried the other way, and this works best for you. The important thing, you have discovered, is to find a routine that works best for you and then to stick to it. Eight in the morning to four in the afternoon is your set routine. You always get up at four. If you have slept badly, then you have a nap just before going to work.

Whatever happens, you try to log eight hours sleep a day. You have heard that most workers on night shift average only 5.6 hours sleep per day. Every day they take little "loans" from their sleep banker. But not you. You know that your dangerously moody sleep banker may call in the loan when you are driving at seventy miles per hour on the freeway. You have heard that 15 percent of night shift workers reported falling asleep driving at least once in three months. You are a survivor. You deposit eight hours in your sleep bank every day.

Your sleep "bank" used to be your bedroom, but you have changed it into a sleeproom. This is the quietest, darkest, most peaceful room with the most comfortable bed in the world. No troubles are allowed in this room—ever. The phone never rings, and you deal firmly and swiftly with any worries, regrets, and guilty feelings that want to keep you awake. Here you can relax.

You lie in bed and slide into your relaxation routine. All troubles leave your mind when your body relaxes. Your foam earplugs muffle all stray sound, your black velvet eyeshade brings you total darkness. You would now suggest sleep to yourself, but you are already drifting off.

Protect your family life

The protection starts with you. You need it. The daytime noise of a family—spouse and two kids—can demolish sleep.

Now if you were sick, the house would be kept quiet for you to sleep during the day. Invalids get what they need. So why not shift workers? You are a "healthy invalid" when it comes to your night shift work sleep needs. So let the family know this. What you are asking for is a fair deal: you help put bread on the table by putting up with the discomforts of shift work, so they give you total quiet for daytime sleep. Have a friendly family meeting about it. The rule here is: Don't rage against noise; organize quiet.

Your organizing starts with the house. Carpeting, acoustic tiles, headphones for the TV and stereo, foam earplugs for you, prizes for quiet kids—whatever works. Your plans will also include the neighborhood. First, let the neighbors know that you are a shift worker. Try to get the kids out of the house as much as possible while you sleep. Trading off day care and baby-sitting with other shift workers can be part of it. If you are a single parent, try to find, or even organize, a support network of others who are in the same boat. Together, you might put together a list of reliable baby-sitters.

Once you have organized your home so that your family is giving you the quiet that you need, it is time to concentrate on their needs. Enjoyable family life doesn't always happen even when you are working days; when you work nights, it takes special effort. Try to organize an hour of quality time with the children every day and schedule regular treats every two weeks, or when days off allow. Organize the good times; don't expect them to happen without effort. There is an old saying about young people: "Youth will be served." One way or another, young people will get the attention that they need. It's better that they get loving attention from you rather than corrective attention from strangers.

Keep your social life alive

Night shift work is probably not as damaging to your social life as evening shift can be, but you still face the same threat of slowly losing touch with your circle of friends. Some of the same solutions therefore apply:

1. Make a timetable of your shifts and let all of your friends have a copy. This helps them schedule you into their social plans and also lets them know that you value their friendship. Also, give out copies to any clubs or societies that you belong to. Most meetings are held in the early part of weekday evenings, which means that you can usually get to them before going on shift. The pressures of shift work may mean cutting down on such meetings, but cutting them all out is probably a mistake. Don't let shift work threaten your social life.

2. Make an effort. Keep in touch with friends as much as you can. Accept invitations to dinners, barbecues, and parties even if you have to leave at 10:00 P.M. to get ready to go on shift. This, of course, means that you will not be drinking anything stronger than tomato juice, but memories of the party will brighten up your shift, and you will keep in touch this way.

How to have night shift security

If you are a woman night shift worker, getting to work, especially on public transit, can be a problem. The best solution is to travel in groups. Your problems are not as bad as those of evening shift workers, who travel an hour later and who leave a workplace where they may have been exposed to troublemakers who could follow or lie in wait for them.

If you are a night shift worker leaving family at home, your peace of mind on shift will depend on knowing that your home is secure. Your three main concerns should be your doors and windows, your phone, and fire.

Doors and windows should be latched and secure so that anyone trying to get in has to break something and make a noise. You can't make a fortress out of your home, but you can make it impossible for anyone to break in quietly. A noisy alarm system is a good idea, especially if there are neighbors who are part of a "block watch" organization. A ringing doorbell should, of course, be ignored at night. If it persists, phone the police and neighbors.

The phone is probably best answered at night by the answering machine. Leave it on the one-ring setting, with a "no one can come to the phone right now . . . " message in a man's voice. In that way your family can identify the caller before making any response. The main thing is to avoid letting anyone know that a lone woman or young people are alone in the house. An answering machine to field all calls can prevent someone's being woken by the phone and blurting out, "No, my parent/husband is on night shift" before being fully awake.

While you are working on night shift, a pager is a good way to make sure that all calls from home reach you immediately. You can set up your own code system, so that 111 means "All's well," 222 means "Phone home when you get the chance," 333 means "Phone home at once," and so on.

Fire at home while you are on night shift should be your third major concern. The threat from fire is sometimes greater than the threat from intruders. There are three main areas to think about: fire prevention, fire detection, and a fire situation plan. Contact your local fire department and use their expert advice on preventing fires and using smoke detectors. Then make sure that everyone at home knows what to do in case of fire. Knowing that your family is as secure from fire as you can make them will help remove stress from your night shift.

How to survive night shift

It's bad enough having trouble sleeping during the day, but dozing off on night shift can be disastrous or even deadly. If you are a nurse, a nuclear power plant operator, an air traffic controller, or an airline pilot, you have the type of job that usually calls for constant alertness. Any failure of alertness can be life threatening to you or to the people you serve. But even on jobs that demand less alertness than these, nodding off can cause major problems. What to do?

The immediate solutions are defensive. Pay attention to every detail in the earlier parts of this book to make sure you get good sleep during the day. Then when you go on shift, think very hard about the lowest point of your body clock cycle, between 3:00 and 6:00 A.M.—The most deadly hours of the graveyard shift. If you have any control over your work scheduling, plan to have the least demands on your alertness in these hours. Get an alarm wrist watch and set it to warn you about the start of these hours of minimum alertness. Finally, try to get a nap in somewhere during the shift. Remember, "Nap and survive; nod off and perish."

The longer-term solutions are offensive: fighting for your rights. What kind of a shift system do you have? How does it rate? All night shift work, but especially high-stress jobs, deserve the very best shift systems, with more than usual time off. You should have a right to take a nap on shift and have a proper time and place for it; workers in Sweden have these rights. The Argentine government rates fifty-two minutes of any night work as equal to sixty minutes of day work. In Israel, night shifts are limited to seven hours. The U.S. lacks a national policy on shift work and in this lags behind many countries. So don't suffer bad working conditions in silence. If no one ever went after better working conditions, steelworkers would still be working eighty-four hour weeks—and so might you.

12

Irregular shifts:
five ways to survive the
toughest shifts of all

A thirty-nine-year-old trucker driving a 1982 White tractor pulling an empty trailer was traveling west on NC 55, eighteen miles west of New Bern, North Carolina, on Monday, June 13, 1988 at 6:30 P.M. The weather was clear, bright, sunny, and dry. Traveling at an estimated 55 miles per hour on level roadway, the truck approached a gentle curve to the left, which continued for seven hundred feet. But the driver did not make the turn into the curve.

Instead, the fifty-two-thousand-pound truck and trailer continued straight ahead. It crossed the right shoulder, entered a roadside ditch, plowed ahead, hit a dirt embankment, crossed a private drive, and having traveled 101 feet from where it left the roadway, struck and broke a twenty-two-inch diameter tree, rolled another sixty-five feet, and came to rest in an open field. No other vehicle was involved. There were no skid marks on the roadway.

The tractor was destroyed. The impact pushed in the firewall on the driver's side about twenty inches. The driver, wearing a lap-shoulder seat belt, was crushed and died at once from "multiple trauma," particularly massive head injuries.

The driver had been employed by the truck owners for about seventeen years and had been a regular driver of heavy trucks for over twelve years. He held a valid North Carolina Class A driver's license with no restrictions. For seven years before the accident, his record showed no traffic convictions or accidents.

He had been on duty ten and a half hours before the accident and drove about half of this time; he was therefore in compliance with hours-of-service regulations. His blood samples showed no drugs or alcohol when tested to National Transportation Safety Board (NTSB) standards. Blood samples were also tested at the request of the state of North Carolina, also with negative results. For much of the weekend before this accident, he had been away from home at church-related functions. Though he normally slept about seven hours a night, he had slept only five hours (2:00 A.M. to 7:00 A.M.) the night before the accident that killed him. The NTSB determined that the probable cause of the accident was the impairment of the truck driver due to fatigue.

This accident shows how deadly fatigue can be even for a day shift worker. This driver was young and experienced and had an exemplary work record. He was using no drugs or alcohol, working steady day shifts, and driving under ideal conditions.

If lack of sleep can be lethal even under such ideal work conditions, how much more dangerous it is for workers sleeping at irregular hours, often far from home, and probably under pressure to work when they are tired.

In the next section you will get a clear picture of just how great these dangers are. The remaining section of this chapter will show you how to deal with these dangers.

The lethal sleep problems of irregular shifts: can you survive them?

Why is it that in the U.S. five truck drivers per week die in accidents, mainly due to fatigue? Why do airline pilots, in survey after survey, rank fatigue as their number-one problem? Why are the sleep problems of irregular shift workers so bad?

Most irregular shift work happens in the transportation industry. It is difficult and costly to organize an orderly shift system to relieve the crews of trucks, trains, and aircraft, who often end their shifts far from home and in a different time zone. Work in all these branches of the transportation industry can mean similar sleep problems. Sleep may be interrupted or delayed by bad weather, machinery breakdowns, or changes in schedule due to unexpected changes in demands for service. Adding to these sleep problems is the stress common to all transportation industry workers. Being in control of a moving machine, whether it is a ship, a train, a jet aircraft, or a truck, is stressful; dozing off can be disastrous.

In a major study, the National Transportation Safety Board found that 31 percent of truck driver fatalities were probably due to fatigue. The Aviation Safety Reporting System, which encourages pilots to make anonymous reports about threats to safety, announced that in 1980, 21 percent of those reports were related to fatigue.

In a similar British study, one-third of the confidential reports by eight hundred pilots mentioned the problem of fatigue caused by a demanding work schedule. Pilots reported that entire crews on long-distance flights had fallen asleep at the controls.

Survivors use good judgment

A small cargo plane was on a low-level return flight to Britain at night over the English Channel when the pilot fell asleep. The right landing gear was ripped off when the plane hit the water. The pilot, startled awake, made a skillful recovery and later made a successful emergency landing.

This incident reminded me of a sign I once saw in small airfield crew room:

"A superior pilot uses his superior judgment to avoid those situations where he might have to use his superior skill."

This pilot's judgment about his fatigue level was not superior, and so he had to rely on his superior skill (and luck) to recover from a desperate situation. For "pilot" you could read "truck driver," "bus driver," and many other skilled transportation workers.

Superior judgment to recognize potentially dangerous situations is especially important for irregular shift workers. The entry into situations where you are expected to control a truck, bus, train, plane, or ship when you should really be getting some sleep may at first appear quite harmless. The dangers appear later. It is therefore important to recognize the entry points early on.

Using superior judgment to avoid dangerous situations

You are fatigued and you know that you should not be driving/ flying/steering. But the boss, or dispatcher, or operations chief, or whoever gives you your orders, asks you to work, and then says:

"I wouldn't normally ask you, but we are in a squeeze."

"There's no one else but you."

"Just this once."

"You help me out on this one and I won't forget it."

"Don't let me down."

"Everyone bends the regulations."

"Pitching in like this is really part of the job."

"You're a hard-working person; you want to get ahead."

"Promotions go to problem solvers."

"If you can't deliver it's gonna cost the company big bucks."

"It's a very competitive world out there."

"You really seem to be a stickler for the regulations."

"This could cost you plenty."

"If you don't want to do things our way, there's others who will."

"Have it your own way, fella."

But it's not just the boss who can put pressure on you; the pressure can come from inside your head:

"I like my boss; I want to please him/her," you may say to yourself. Or:

"I'm a tough, problem-solving, can-do professional; let's go!"

"I've worked other times when I've been tired, and survived."

"I can do it—just this once."

"I need the money."

"Everyone else does it."

"If I don't go along now, I will get the dirty jobs later."

"I can handle fatigue. I've got some 'pink hearts' and 'cross-tops' to keep me awake."

How to avoid entry into risky situations

The pressures to give in to what the boss wants can be real and strong. The boss may be a senior staffer who drove a truck or flew a plane when you were just a little kid. It is hard to stand up to that kind of clout. But the pressures can be just as strong when they come from inside your own head. How can you avoid them?

The simple answer is this: Be prepared. Think about the situation carefully, before you are under pressure, and come to a firm decision then. Take a hard look at the persuasive arguments. Most of them boil down to this: you are being pressured to risk your neck (and possibly to break the law) by working when you are fatigued. It is strange fact that bosses who would never ask you to work when you are sick or injured sometimes expect you to work when you are fatigued.

What is really at stake if you refuse to work when you are fatigued? Make yourself a list:

1. You'll incur your boss's displeasure or anger.

2. The plum jobs, the good routes, may stop coming your way.

3. Promotion may go to a junior rival.

4. Money may be lost.

5. Your job might be on the line, especially if there is a downsizing.

What is at stake if you agree to work when you are fatigued? Make yourself another list:

1. Your license may be suspended or lost.

2. You career may be ended by injury or by crash-related litigation.

3. Your life could be lost. None of the truckers or pilots who crash due to fatigue expect it to happen.

If you say "yes" to your boss's request, it may be because you are assuming that you will have a normal shift and you will manage your fatigue as you have done successfully in the past. But if you run into bad weather, delays, or breakdowns, your fatigue may be the final straw. Accidents are often due to a group of small factors that add up to a deadly total.

Your career is more important than your job, and the risk of death or injury for yourself and many others should outweigh all else. No punishment that your boss can inflict on you can compare with the punishment of a crash.

Survivors use naps

Even though you use your superior judgment to avoid working shifts when you are fatigued, there will nevertheless be times when you are on shift and dead tired. You could decide to keep on working and try to fight off your fatigue, but that could be a gamble with your life, a gamble that five U.S. truck drivers take every week and lose. Or you might decide to use drugs to stay awake, only you remember that after fatigue, drugs were the main cause of fatal accidents to heavy truck drivers according to a National Transportation Safety Board study. So what options are left?

Your superior judgment tells you that you must either abandon the shift altogether or else take a nap. If you were a Swedish worker on night shift, that might not be a problem. Swedish factories and mines have rest rooms with bunks where workers can take naps. But for many irregular shift workers—airline pilots, for instance— naps are forbidden.

A study by NASA and the Federal Aviation Authority showed that naps by pilots during the cruise portion of long flights, when little is happening, improved performance during the critical approach-and-landing portion. Eventually this prohibition on naps may change. In 1989 Boeing revealed plans to introduce alarms to wake up sleeping pilots on long-haul flights. This is a clear recognition of the extent to which pilots do, in fact, nod off on the flight deck.

Naps are probably more important for irregular shift workers than for anyone else. Fighting sleepiness on the job is probably a familiar struggle for you if you work these shifts. If you take a nap you may be breaking regulations or losing time, and when you wake up you may feel groggy for a while. On the other hand, if you don't take a nap the result may be even worse.

To keep working when you are fatigued is a gamble. If you are faced with the choice of this "nod-off-and-crash roulette" or of taking a short, planned nap under safe conditions, your superior judgment will certainly help you make a sensible choice.

The next chapter goes into the subject of napping more fully.

Survivors band together

If you are being asked, or pressured unfairly, to work when you are fatigued, the dispatcher or crew chief has the whole clout of the company behind him or her; what clout do you have? If you stand alone, threatening to quit is the extent of your clout. That is not usually a big threat, unless you are a star performer and hard to replace. If you belong to a union, you have plenty of clout, but the 1980s trend towards deregulation has weakened the power of many unions.

The effect of deregulation has been similar in the trucking and air transportation industries. In each industry, the licensing requirements have been eased, allowing small operators and companies to enter the industries in large numbers. This has often caused fierce competition, leading to price cutting and lowered safety standards. At the same time the federal inspection agencies who are responsible for enforcing safety standards have had their budgets slashed.

Trucking is now a two-tiered industry. On the top tier are company drivers who are paid a flat rate per mile, are given an allowance for loading and unloading time, and enjoy social and health benefits. On the bottom tier are owner-operators, who own, maintain, and usually are making payments on their big trucks. They often have to work very long hours, and they sometimes cut corners, in order to survive.

The airlines also are a two-tiered industry. On the top tier are the major carriers who fly the intercity "hub" routes. The strict Part 121 FAA standards govern these carriers. On the bottom tier are mostly small feeder airlines flying the "spoke" routes into the big city hubs. The less strict Part 135 FAA standards govern these smaller carriers. Many bottom tier carriers run excellent, well-maintained, safe operations, never pressuring their air crews to fly long hours or in marginal conditions. Others are less scrupulous.

Truck drivers and air crews who are in the bottom tier of their industry are the irregular shift workers most likely to be under pressure to work when they are fatigued.

If you drive heavy trucks for a living, it may surprise you to know that in some ways you are better protected against unreasonable hours of work than are airline pilots. Your daily log sheet, in the form of a time chart, shows very clearly the hours that you have spent: off duty, in the truck's sleeper berth, driving, and on duty.

Also, your monthly log summary sheet shows for each day of the month: hours worked (total of driving and on duty), total hours on duty in the last seven days, and hours available to work tomorrow (seventy hours minus the total hours already on duty in the last seven days).

A highway patrol officer inspecting this log can see at a glance the pattern of work and rest that you claim to have followed in the last week and whether you have had enough rest to drive safely.

You may sometimes find your log sheet more of a pain than a protection, especially if you have to spend three days waiting around in a motel miles from home because you have run out of hours. However, few professional drivers would like to see log sheets abolished. The highways are dangerous enough as it is.

If you are an airline pilot, neither you nor your passengers (amazingly) have the protection of the detailed, personal work-and-rest-time log sheets carried by heavy truck drivers. At none of our airports are you, as a pilot about to fly, asked by inspectors to produce a log sheet to show that you are well rested. Each of the thousands of parts of the aircraft that you will fly has a log entry showing that it has been checked for wear and tear. Does it make sense, then, to have no such log for the pilot who will be in command? The no-names, confidential reporting systems for pilots in the U.S and also in Britain show that fatigue is a major concern and problem for pilots. Some pilots believe that a personal daily and monthly log would be an important step to combat pilot fatigue. It could show hours spent: off duty sleeping, off duty awake, commuting, on duty, flying, and on duty during the last seven days.

The pressures on truck drivers and air crews to work when they are tired is just one corner of a much bigger struggle: the unending battle for decent working conditions. To fight this battle you need clout. Clout comes from banding together with your fellow workers. Remember the steelworker who worked twelve-hour shifts seven days a week? If he refused to work these hours, the mill would immediately hire someone who would. Conditions only improved when the steelworkers banded together for better conditions.

Survivors protect their families

Irregular shifts are the toughest of all shift systems on you, the shift worker; they are also the toughest on your family. Anniversaries, birthdays, weekends, Thanksgiving, Passover, Easter, Christmas may be spent in a motel hundreds or thousands of miles from home. The strains that this can place on you and your family are obvious.

All of the ways that regular shift workers must use to protect their family life apply with added force to you. Separation from your partner must be balanced by big blocks of quality time in between trips. Cellular phones mean that you can stay in touch on a daily basis and are available for emergencies. You also need to make extra efforts to keep in contact with your children. When you are far away, phone calls should always include them. You are eating alone at a lunch counter far from home? Write them post cards. Even if you get home before the card is delivered, it shows that you were thinking of them when you were far away. It will also brighten up your lunch break.

Keeping your family life alive when you are far from home will let you sleep better and will help you cope with the stress and fatigue of your job. A strong family life is protective. One of the very important findings of the National Transportation Safety Board inquiry into truck accidents fatal to the driver was:

"A disproportionately high percentage of drivers who used drugs are single, separated, or divorced."

Protect your family life, and it will protect you.

STEP 7

NAP AND SURVIVE: NOD OFF AND PERISH

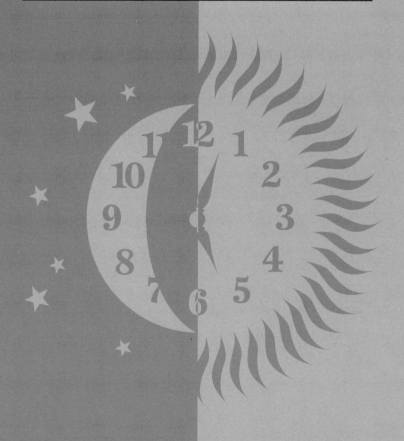

13

Napping is an essential survival skill
—especially for shift workers

I was very drowsy as I drove along the highway at about four in the afternoon in bright sunlight. Keeping my eyes open took a big effort, and sometimes my head nodded forward, bringing my attention back with a snap. I recognized all the signs of the "doze of death." I pulled the car off the highway into a shady spot, made a pillow out of my jacket, looked at my watch, and plunged into a refreshing snooze. Seven minutes later I woke up from this light nap feeling fresh and alert. The last seventy miles of my journey I was wide awake.

Drowsiness is a factor in roughly 200,000 U.S. automobile accidents a year and at least 1,600 fatalities, according to the U.S. Department of Transportation. Few of those accidents would have happened if the drivers involved had pulled over to the roadside and taken a ten-minute nap.

Driving when you are seriously short of sleep may be more dangerous than driving when drunk. Drunk drivers may drive very dangerously, but they will at least try to avoid a crash. A driver who nods off will not make the slightest effort to avoid a head-on crash or to steer away from the edge of a cliff. The accidents of drivers who fall asleep while driving are three times more likely to be fatal than those of drivers who are awake. If sleepy drivers are stopped by the police because of their erratic driving, their condition may not even be recognized. There are Breathalyzers to detect if a vehicle's driver is running on alcohol, but the police are not yet using "sleepalyzers" to detect fatigue.

Falling asleep on the job has resulted in ships going aground, trucks rear-ending school buses, and trains ramming head-on, as you saw in "Shift work dangers: asleep on the job" (Chapter 1). Any of these accidents could have been avoided with a nap.

But what is a nap? In this section a "nap" means just this: A planned, five to twenty minutes, light sleep, under safe conditions while on the job.

The key word here is "planned." A nap is planned and makes you feel better; nodding off is an accident and may be a disaster.

Naps are a very important survival skill for all shift workers, but are particularly essential for nurses, truck drivers, pilots, and other irregular shift workers.

In choosing to take such naps to avoid accidentally dozing off, these workers display superior judgment, because they might otherwise enter situations from which even their superior skill might not be able to save them.

Naps are natural

Your normal sleep is made up of five ninety-minute "naps." In these ninety-minute cycles you take about half an hour to plunge down into the stage of deep sleep, where you remain for about forty-five minutes before coming up for ten or fifteen minutes of REM sleep. This rapid-eyeball-movement sleep is filled with dreams from which you are easily aroused. If all is well, you plunge back down again into another ninety-minute cycle.

You will remember from Chapter 2 that for our ancestors, as well as for wild animals, being asleep could be very dangerous. In a tribe of prehistoric humans or a herd of antelope where sleep is taken in short naps, there will always be one or two members awake to sound the alarm if predators are around.

So sleeping under difficult or even dangerous conditions is normal for all creatures, including us. Short, refreshing naps during safe, slack periods at work make good sense; naps are natural.

Nevertheless, naps tend to have a bad name. They have come to be associated with the daytime sleep of children and seniors. Mature adults don't need naps, goes this mistaken thinking. To be "caught napping" is shameful.

It certainly is shameful and, more importantly, dangerous to accidentally fall asleep on the job. It is precisely to prevent this happening that you should take a planned, short nap, under safe conditions, while on the job. When you do this, you will be in good company. Intelligent napping has meant survival to many people in the past.

One of history's most famous nappers was Winston Churchill, Britain's prime minister during the second World War. Here is how he described his daily nap schedule in his book *The Gathering Storm*:

"I always went to bed for at least one hour as early as possible in the afternoon and exploited to the full my happy gift of falling almost immediately to sleep. By this means I was able to press a day and a half's work into one."

Napoleon was able to take a nap even during battles. He compared his thinking to the opening and closing of drawers in a cabinet, each containing a particular subject. When he wished to sleep, the owner of this powerful mind just "closed all the drawers."

Leonardo da Vinci, though, may have been history's champion napper. His schedule was fifteen minutes of sleep every four hours— nonstop. Leonardo, among the greatest of all painters, architects, and scientists, was able to sustain his genius on naps only.

Napping on the job

Leonardo's incredible sleep schedule fascinated a sleep researcher named Claudio Stampi. Fifteen minutes of sleep every four hours means a total of only ninety minutes sleep in twenty-four hours, or one and a half hours sleep per day. Could anyone really survive on so little sleep? Stampi found a twenty-seven-year-old artist who was willing to be an experimental subject and reduce his sleep from a normal eight hours per night down to thirty minutes every four hours. This was a less severe version of Leonardo's schedule, but it still gave the young artist only three hours sleep in twenty-four.

The artist remained on this schedule under Stampi's observation for three weeks. Like Leonardo, he found that this routine allowed him to get more work done, and so he volunteered to remain on it for another two months.

This experiment indicated that it is possible to function on nothing but naps, but it did not show if the artist was wide awake and able to work efficiently between naps. The quality and volume of the artist's work before going on this schedule and during it were not measured.

How could the quality of work done by a napping worker be accurately measured? An answer was found outside the laboratory. Stampi found a ready-made experiment to measure the quality of various types of napping. The "experiment" was a solo yacht race and the "laboratory" was the Atlantic Ocean. The sleep problem for the sailors in this race looked like this:

You are alone in a small sailboat, sailing in a three-thousand-mile race across the Atlantic Ocean. Doing well in this race is not good enough for you; you want to win it. A cash prize and valuable endorsements for the sponsor's products could be yours.

You will have to sail with great skill to win. You will have to respond quickly to changes in wind and sea conditions to squeeze the last drop of performance out of your sailboat. You also have to avoid collision, day and night, with other sailboats, with giant freighters, and with rocks and sand banks.

Sleep is one of your greatest problems. Since there is no one else to help you, how will you stay alert day after day without a good sleep? How can you be sure that you won't be asleep or just dozing off when you are on a collision course with another competitor or when the sharp bow of a giant freighter comes out of the mist like a huge steel knife?

In 1980, the fifty-four yachtsmen competing in the Observer

Single-Handed Transatlantic Race (OSTAR) faced these problems in sailing from Plymouth, England, to Newport, Rhode Island, along one of the world's busiest ocean highways.

Stampi recognized that participation in this contest meant solving very tough sleep problems. It was an experiment with risks and rewards that no laboratory could match. The fifty-four yachtsmen agreed to keep sleep logs for Stampi during the race. The results of this survey were quite revealing; they showed:

1. The fastest crossing took seventeen days; the slowest took forty-nine days.

2. Those who took the shortest naps (between twenty minutes and one hour) were the fastest sailors.

3. The total amount of daily sleep taken by the best-performing sailors ranged between 3 and 5.5 hours, with the highest speeds being achieved by those sleeping 4.5 hours per day.

4. Total daily sleep time could be reduced by 60 percent to 70 percent without harming performance.

5. Even naps as short as ten minutes were beneficial. This minimum length for a useful nap confirmed the findings of earlier research, according to Stampi.

The total freedom of these sailors to nap or sleep whenever they wanted was an important feature of this study. It was up to them to decide on the sleep schedule that would be most effective in racing across the Atlantic Ocean.

Airline pilots flying the Atlantic are far less free regarding naps; Federal Aviation Authority (FAA) regulations forbid them. Yet the need for pilots' freedom to take naps is clear and obvious. A pilot could take a short nap during the normally uneventful mid-Atlantic portion of the crossing while the plane is on autopilot and the copilot monitors the flight deck. He or she would then be rested and refreshed for the busy and demanding final approach and landing stages of the flight.

A report by Graeber and Curtis for the National Aeronautic and

Space Administration (NASA) and the FAA described a study of nine volunteer Boeing 747 crews who were allowed to take naps during forty minutes of the cruise part of long flights. The study showed improved performance during the final stages of these flights.

The downside of napping as far as air crews are concerned is that when it is finally permitted by FAA regulations, it may be used as a way of reducing rest time between flights by aggressive, cost-cutting managers. Every silver lining has a cloud.

The beneficial effects of having sleeping facilities at the job site and allowing naps during shift work has long been recognized in many countries. Workers in Swedish factories and mines have rest rooms where they can take naps during night shifts. In Denmark, half of the policemen in one survey took short naps during night shift. In Japan, between 40 percent and 50 percent of night shift workers take naps.

The right to take short naps during slack periods while on shift has much to recommend it. Shift workers were once denied the right to have lunch breaks, coffee breaks, and even bathroom breaks. These rights are now a fixed part of decent working conditions. Taking short naps during night shifts should now be added to these basic rights. There is little doubt that safety, efficiency, goodwill, and productivity would be improved by such a change.

How to nap

Knowing how to take a nap and then taking one when you need it is every bit as much a survival skill as knowing how to drive a car or knowing emergency first aid. Any skill that can save you from the "doze-of-death" at work or on the highway is a skill that you must have.

Here are some key points in survival napping:

1. Nap ruthlessly: If you are very thirsty and you really need water, I mean YOU REALLY NEED WATER, you will get it; nothing will stand in your way. Or if your breathing is cut off,

you will struggle fiercely to restore it; again, nothing will stand in your way. We are talking here about vital necessities; we are talking about survival. You will be ruthless in getting what you need. This is the way you must be about taking a nap when you need it; you must be ruthless. This means that any person or thing that stands in the way of your nap gets very quietly but very firmly pushed aside.

2. Nap securely: When you sleep anywhere you are at your most helpless and need to be sure of your security. This is especially important when you take a nap away from your home. The best security is to have someone with you who can wake you if need be. If you nap alone in a car or truck, be sure the doors are locked and activate your alarm system if you have one. If you are a woman driver, getting one of these alarm systems is more than just a good idea.

3. Avoid sleep debt: Try to avoid going short of your regular sleep, hoping to catch up with a nap. Keep your sleep debt paid up. If you are short of your vital deep sleep when you take a nap, your body will grab that deep sleep while it can. Your body plays for keeps. This means that you will plunge into a deep sleep and wake up feeling groggy with "sleep inertia." This sleep inertia may reduce your efficiency for several minutes, which could be a problem if you are a nurse, a pilot, a firefighter, or anyone who has to respond quickly and effectively to emergencies. Deep sleep "will not be denied," say sleep researchers, so avoid a sleep debt.

4. Pick the right nap length: When you take a nap your body doesn't know that this is only a nap, and so it enters your normal ninety-minute sleep cycle. If your nap ends when you are in the deep sleep stage, you will wake up feeling groggy with sleep inertia. To avoid this, nap for less than twenty minutes.

5. Set your alarm: If you want to take a short, planned sleep, or

nap, you need a wake-up call of some kind. You certainly want to avoid having your nap stretch out into a (possibly disastrous) sleep. To make sure that this doesn't happen, get a digital watch with an alarm function, or a pocket alarm clock. If you don't have an alarm with you, you can try napping in a sitting-up position so that when you fall asleep and your head nods forward, you wake up. However, this means having a very short nap, or series of naps, and although these can be very refreshing, you can relax better with your alarm set. Some truck drivers take a nap while holding a lighted cigarette between their fingers and wake up when it burns them. An alarm clock is more reliable and easier on the fingers.

6. Nap proudly, nap often: Never be ashamed to take a nap any more than you are ashamed to breathe. Start watching for nap opportunities. While others take a fifteen-minute coffee break, you can take a ten minute nap. Somebody is driving you somewhere? Catch a few z's. Waiting for a flight at an airport? Set your alarm and freshen up with a nap. The more you practice grabbing odd moments of time to take naps, the better you will get. Always keep in mind the difference between taking a nap and dozing off: a nap is something that you decide to take; dozing off is something that takes you.

Summary

Forty Sleep Problems and Solutions for Shift Workers

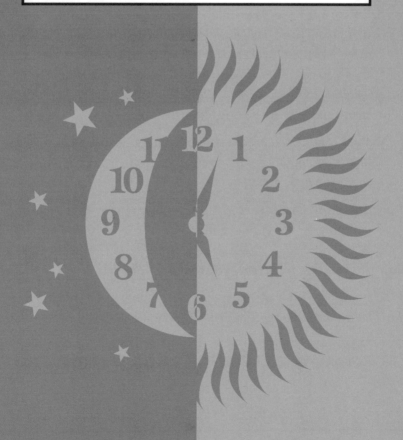

Turn to the list below whenever you recognize that lack of sleep is affecting your life. You'll find concise answers to common problems that many shift workers face.

1. **Problem:** Why can't I sleep? What is a good "rule-of-thumb" about sleep problems?

   Solution: Sleep is like healing. If you have an injury, you remove all of the things that prevent healing, like dirt and bacteria. Then leave the rest to your body. It is very smart; it knows how to heal. It's the same with sleep. Your main effort is to remove all of the things that prevent sleep, like noise, heavy meals, and worries. Then leave the rest to your body. It is very smart. It knows how to sleep.

The problem can be lethal

2. **Problem:** What is the best way to tackle sleep problems?

   Solution: Recognize that these problems are serious. They can grind your health down slowly or kill you quickly in asleep-at-the-wheel accidents. Solving them is survival skill that you can learn. Start with the easy things first.

The problem may be one for your doctor

3. **Problem:** Tired all the time. Fatigue always seems to be a bigger problem for you than it does for fellow shift workers in your age group.

   Solution: Check over the symptoms in Step 2. Your problem may be one for your doctor.

Fix the easy things first: your sleeproom

4. **Problem:** Wide awake in bed. You do not sleep well in your bedroom although nothing seems to be wrong with it.

   Solution: Your bedroom should be a sleeproom where nothing happens except sex and sleep. Remove ringing phones, TV, computers, work/study materials, worries, arguments, and problems of all descriptions. Your sleeproom must be a refuge from the world; keep out intruders of all kinds.

5. **Problem:** Household noise disturbs your sleep.

   Solution: Don't rage against noise; organize quiet. Have a family meeting, explain what shift work is like, and ask for help. Ideas: TV headphones, acoustic tiles, earplugs, rewards for quiet kids, baby-sitters, move to house with basement rec room.

6. **Problem:** Neighborhood noise disturbs your sleep.

   Solution: Again, don't rage against noise; organize quiet. Visit neighbors and ask for help. Leave shift timetable and follow-up thank-you notes. Join local antinoise groups. If all else fails, move. Survival may demand strong measures.

7. **Problem:** Stomach upset. Shift work gives you digestive upsets like constipation and heartburn that keep you awake.

   Solution: Avoid greasy, fried, fast, and junk foods. Eat lots of veggies and fruit. Give your stomach light work to do while you sleep; it will thank you by letting you sleep peacefully.

8. **Problem:** Couch potato. Your job needs little physical effort, and lack of exercise has made you overweight, but shift work seems to give you time to do little besides work and sleep.

   Solution: Regular exercise is an essential part of your shift work survival skills. An important advantage of shift work is that it often allows you to schedule uncrowded daytime activity in many places, including sport/exercise clubs. If all else fails, fifteen or twenty minutes jogging a day can give you the exercise that you need for good health, better sleep, and better sex.

9. **Problem:** Love life fade-out. Shift work has had a bad effect on your sex and love life.

   Solution: Talk this over with your partner. Schedule prime time for your love life and give it first place, ahead of television, parties, alcohol, shopping, and even golf. If shift work continues to damage your love life, survival may mean updating your resume and searching for a less damaging job.

A hard look at drugs

10. **Problem:** Sleeping pills. Should you take them to sleep better between shifts?

    Solution: Sleeping pills do not bring normal sleep. Doctors advise against continuous use. You use crutches only while your broken leg mends, not all the time. Use sleeping pills the same way. Save them for rare emergencies.

11. **Problem:** Sleeping pills. You use them regularly, but they don't work as well as they did, and you often feel tired.

    Solution: Unless your doctor insists that you take them, quit. You may need your doctor's help and supervision to do this if you are a longtime user.

12. **Problem:** Coffee. You take a long time to go to sleep after a shift and don't seem to get enough rest. You drink four or five mugs of coffee on shift to stay awake.

    Solution: Cut way back on your coffee breaks; you will sleep better and not need that coffee to stay awake.

13. **Problem:** Nightcap. After a shift you find that beer or liquor helps you to get to sleep, but that your sleep is not long or restful.

    Solution: Alcohol can bring unconsciousness, but not normal healthy sleep. Reduce then eliminate nightcaps as soon as you can.

14. **Problem:** "Uppers." To stay awake on shift or to drive your big truck long hours to meet a delivery deadline you sometimes take amphetamines or methamphetamines ("speed," "cross-tops," "pink hearts," "black beauties," etc.). These drugs produce bad sleep and wild dreams when you stop taking them.

    Solution: Quit while you are ahead. Studies connect the use of these drugs with many fatal accidents. "Speed freaks" do not belong on our highways.

Dealing with the sleep wreckers in your mind

15. **Problem:** Worries. Worries about the future, regrets about the past, or guilt about things that you did or didn't do often keep you awake.

    Solution: Put these sleep wreckers under a bright light and if you see any action needed, decide to take it. If not, put them in the garbage can. Then go to sleep.

16. **Problem:** Workaholic. You bring your job home, take it to bed with you, and often dream that you are at work. However, you don't get good sleep (or overtime pay) for working those "shifts."

    Solution: Start switching your job "off" an hour before you go to bed. Even ten minutes watching a soothing National Geographic special on TV will help. Never think or talk about your job in your sleeproom.

17. **Problem:** It's quiet and comfortable but you're wide awake. You are lying in bed, wide awake, and you must get some sleep.

    Solution: Make your own "sleeping pill" with suggestion. First, relax your body thoroughly. Now make yourself a sleeping pill out of words like "sleep," "slumber," "doze," and "dream." Take your homemade "pill" as often as needed.

18. **Problem:** Suggestion. Will it work for me?

    Solution: Say the word "yawn" to yourself three times. Presto, you yawned! Suggestion works for you. Suggestion has enormous, gentle power. The whole advertising industry is built on the use of suggestion.

19. **Problem:** Junk thinking. You are lying in bed, wide awake, and you must get some sleep, but your head is crowded with unruly thoughts.

    Solution: Time to reach for the "cosmic vacuum cleaner." This imaginary vacuum cleaner has a hose that is connected to a black hole in space. Black holes swallow anything that comes near them—planets, stars, even galaxies; nothing is too big for a black hole to gobble up. So the cosmic vacuum cleaner can swallow any of your stray thoughts, however big they are. Just one pass with the cosmic vacuum cleaner and, Pfit! they're gone. Even thoughts of your friends and family shouldn't be keeping you awake, so Pfit! they're gone too. Now you can sleep.

Dealing with special problems of shift work

20. **Problem:** Shift changes bring sleep troubles. When your shift system rotates, it always moves you to the shift before, or anticlockwise. For instance, you move from morning shift to night shift. You find it very hard to get used to the new shift times, and by the time you do, it is time to change again.

    Solution: Your troubles come from an old-fashioned shift system. Research has shown that when shifts rotate forward (from night shift to morning shift, for example) your "body clock" gets used to the change far quicker and you sleep better. Shift rotation clockwise is body-clock-wise. Talk to your union; talk to your boss. If all else fails, update your resume and look for an employer who has a modern shift system.

21. **Problem:** A "morning person" on night shifts. You find it almost impossible to get used to night shift, even if you are on night shift all the time.

    Solution: You may be a "lark," or "morning person." For larks, morning is the best time of day; they wake up without an alarm clock and very much dislike working at unusual times. If you are 100 percent lark you may never get used to night shifts and may have to give them up.

22. **Problem:** Rapid shift changes. Although your shifts rotate clockwise (night shift to morning shift, etc.) you are just settling in to a shift when it's time to change again.

    Solution: Your body clock is delicate and takes time to get used to a shift change. Change should either be slow, with more than twenty shifts before a change, so that you get used to it, or very fast, with less than three shifts in a row, so that it's all over before your body clock gets upset.

23. **Problem:** A new shift system, is it good or bad? Your shift system may be changed, but it is hard to tell whether the changes will be good or bad and in what ways.

    Solution: You need some way of comparing the new system with the one you are used to. Turn to the "Sleep and Shift Work" section of this book, where you will find "How to rate your own shift system." This will give you the help you need.

24. **Problem:** To bed late, up early. You get home from your evening shift after 1:00 A.M., and you are lucky to be asleep by 1:30 or 2:00 A.M., but you still want to get up at 6:00 A.M. to put breakfast on the table and see the kids off to school. Then it's hard to get back to sleep.

    Solution: Don't try. Your body clock is going to switch on your morning energy surge while you are trying to get back to sleep. So stay up and nap in the afternoon just before going on shift, when your body clock is turning your energy down.

25. **Problem:** You hardly ever see your family. You are at work during evening family time. You get home when they are asleep and get up after they have gone to school.

    Solution: You have to make the times that you do see them count. Whether it's breakfast or your days off, make it quality time. Explain to the kids exactly what shift work is and make a timetable showing when you will have days off. Involve them in planning your day-off time with them.

26. **Problem:** Evening shifts are making you into a grouch. When you see the kids at breakfast, you are sleepy, and it often turns into a complaint session.

    Solution: Accentuate the positive. Find out what is going well for them and talk about it. Encourage them. Children thrive on praise. Reasonable limits on noise, homework, and coming home on time can be set and held with good-humored firmness.

27. **Problem:** Evening shifts still threaten your family life. You have tried everything, but your family life is still suffering from the effects of you being on evening shifts.

    Solution: Try to get moved to days, but if that fails, begin to look for work elsewhere. Your family is worth more than any job. Update your resume and job hunt. A big advantage of evening shift is that it leaves your days free to do this.

28. **Problem:** Your social life dies due to evening shifts. Your social life is fading away since you have been on evening shift. Friends no longer expect you to be available and don't bother anymore to ask you to a party, barbecue, or bowling.

    Solution: Make copies of your shift timetable for the next month or two and give them to all of your friends and any clubs or groups you belong to. This will let them know when you are able to join in the fun, and more importantly, it will let them know that you value their friendship and want to maintain it.

29. **Problem:** The shift work ghetto. Nobody understands what it's like being on shift work.

    Solution: Other shift workers understand. It's good to have a buddy from your workplace in any job; in shift work it's practically a necessity. Cultivate a shift work buddy whom you can talk freely with after work or over the phone. Unwinding like this reduces job stress, especially after a tough shift, and will help you sleep better.

30. **Problem:** The workplace and the commute home can be dangerous for you, especially if you are a woman. You can be threatened while you work, when you leave work, or in parking lots, deserted streets, or public transit late at night.

    Solution: Shift work brings enough sleep-destroying stresses without this too. This calls for group action from fellow employees, with whom you can organize support groups, car pools, and escorts.

31. **Problem:** Intruders. While on evening or night shift, you worry about the safety of your family from intruders. Anxiety about the safety of those at home adds to the other stresses of shift work.

    Solution: Those at home should not open the door to any unknown caller or reveal on the phone that you are not there. A pager or cellular phone at work can keep you closely in touch with home.

32. **Problem:** Fire. While on evening or night shift you worry about fire at home.

    Solution: Contact your local fire department about fire prevention, fire detection, and a good fire situation plan. Make sure the whole family is fire-safety conscious.

33. **Problem:** Nodding off driving home. You have often almost nodded off while driving home.

    Solution: Nodding off at the wheel kills about 1,600 Americans each year. If any of these drivers had pulled over for a ten-minute nap, they would be alive today. It's better to get home ten minutes late than to risk the "doze-of-death."

34. **Problem:** Nodding off on night shift. Your job demands that you are alert on night shift; nodding off could be a disaster.

    Solution: The time when you are most likely to nod off on night shift is between 3:00 and 6:00 A.M. During this period your body clock turns your energy down to its lowest for the day. Try to schedule your night shift work so that the least demanding and responsible work is done then. Fit in a nap if you can. A 10- or 15-minute nap can work wonders as long as you are not exhausted. Use a watch with an alarm function to keep your nap within limits.

35. **Problem:** Unfair pressure to work. Your boss puts a lot of pressure on you to work extra hours. This pressure can be hard to resist, especially if you need the money, you are worried about job security, and you are not tired at the time you are being pressured.

    Solution: Be prepared for the pressure. Think about the risks you are being asked to take by working when you are exhausted, and make your decision calmly. If you refuse to work, remember that no punishment your boss can hand out is worse than the punishment of an accident at work.

36. **Problem:** Why refuse work? You can handle your fatigue. You have worked when you were exhausted before and know how to handle it, so why not keep doing it?

    Solution: You may be expecting your shift to be a normal one, as before. But if you run into unexpected troubles, your fatigue may be the last straw. Accidents are often due to a lot of little problems that add up to a deadly total.

37. **Problem:** Naps make you feel groggy. You can take naps on shift, but sometimes you wake up feeling really groggy and it takes twenty or thirty minutes before you are working properly.

    Solution: Follow the rules of napping:

    1. Use naps for tune-ups only. Get your regular sleep.

    2. Even a nap as short as ten minutes is valuable.

    3. Ideal nap length is ten to twenty minutes.

    4. Use a watch with an alarm to nap within limits.

38. **Problem:** How can you work at maximum and sleep at minimum for ten days? You must stay awake as much as possible to finish a job in ten days. You are mostly free to sleep or nap whenever you want. What is the most efficient sleep or nap plan for you to follow?

    Solution: It is possible for some people to work efficiently on only four to five hours total sleep per day. They do this by taking their sleep in ten-to-twenty-minute naps. In a single-handed sailboat race across the Atlantic, one of the sailors slept like this for ten days. He experienced no bad effects, and one very good effect: he won the race. His competitors who "napped" for two, three, and up to seven hours did poorly.

39. **Problem:** Overtime pressure. You are under heavy pressure to work many overtime shifts, often at very short notice. These shifts are upsetting your family life and your sleep.

    Solution: You have lots of company. Many businesses now prefer to make their staff work overtime rather than hire extra untrained help. Changing this is probably beyond your power; the solutions are in collective action, which means collective bargaining by a union. One solution is for workers to be able to "bank" overtime and take time off when they have accumulated a week.

40. **Problem:** Wide awake in your sleeproom. You have tried everything to bring sleep and you are still lying in bed wide awake.

    Solution: Get up and leave your sleeproom. It's not a toss-and-turn room. Then do some monotonous chores that you have been putting off, like cleaning out a cupboard or working on your taxes. Avoid "rewarding" yourself with a snack. It won't be long before you are yawning and returning to your sleeproom.

Shift work and upset sleep schedules can bring problems, but these problems do have solutions. Tackle them one at a time, starting as this book did with the easy ones, and then move on to the tough ones. You will find that as your sleep improves, so will your work and your whole outlook on life.

REFERENCES

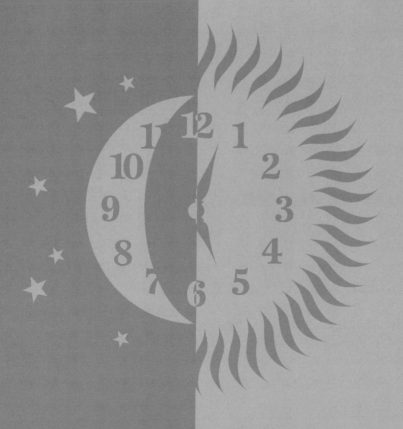

Ashton, H. "Guidelines for the Rational Use of Benzodiazepines." *Drugs*, 48, no. 1 (1994): 25–40.

Ashton, C. H., and Edwards, C. "Which Drug? (3) Hypnotics." *Pharmaceutical Journal* (1991): 702–704.

Clare, A. "Chairman's Summing Up." In Freeman, H. and Y. Rue. *The Benzodiazepines in Current Clinical Practice*. Royal Society of Medicine Services International Congress and Symposium Series no. 114. London: Royal Society of Medicine Services Ltd., 1987.

Coleman, R. M. "Shiftwork Scheduling for the 1990s." *Personnel*. (January 1989): 10–15.

Czeisler, C. A., et al. "Bright Light Resets the Human Circadian Pacemaker Independent of the Timing of the Sleep-Wake Cycle." *Science* 233 (1986): 667–71.

Czeisler, C. A., M. C. Moore-Ede, R. M. Coleman. "Rotating Shift Work Schedules That Disrupt Sleep Are Improved by Applying Circadian Principles." *Science* 217 (1982):460–62.

Folkard, S. and T. H. Monk, eds. *Hours of Work*. New York: John Wiley & Sons, 1985.

Freeman, H. and Y. Rue. *The Benzodiazepines in Current Clinical Practice*. Royal Society of Medicine Services International Congress and Symposium Series no. 114. London: Royal Society of Medicine Services Ltd, 1987.

Green, R. and R. Skinner. *The Log. British Airline Pilot's Association Monthly Journal* (October 1987).

Hartmann, E. *The Sleeping Pill*. New Haven: Yale University Press, 1978.

Horne, J. "Stay Awake, Stay Alive!" *New Scientist* (January 4, 1992): 20–24.

Interchurch World Movement. *Report on the Steel Strike of 1919*. New York: Harcourt Brace, 1920.

Joscelyn, K. B. and A. C. Donelson. "The Identification of Drugs of Interest." In *Highway Safety*. National Highway Traffic Safety Administration Report no. DOT HS-805-299, *Drugs Research Methodology*, vol. 2. Washington, D.C.: U.S. Department of Transportation, 1980. Reprinted in Rothe, J. P. *The Trucker's World: Risk, Safety and Mobility*. New Brunswick: Transaction Publishers, 1991.

Kogi, K. "Introduction to the Problems of Shiftwork." In Folkard, S., and T. H. Monk, eds. *Hours of Work*. New York: John Wiley & Sons, 1985.

Lauber, J. K., and P. J. Kayten. "Sleepiness, Circadian Dysrhythmia, and Fatigue in Transportation Accidents." *Sleep* 11, no. 6 (1988): 503–12.

Lund, Adrian, et.al. "Drug Use by Tractor Trailer Drivers." *Journal of Forensic Sciences* (Sept. 198). Reprinted in Rothe, J. P. *The Trucker's World: Risk, Safety and Mobility*. New Brunswick: Transaction Publishers, 1991.

McKim, W. A. *Drugs and Behavior*. Englewood Cliffs: Prentice Hall, 1986.

Moog, R. "Optimization of Shiftwork." *Ergonomics* 30 no. 9 (1987): 1249–59.

Moore-Ede, M. "Shift Workers at Greater Risk for Morbidity." *Patient Care* 23 (1989): 27–29.

Nance, J. J. *Blind Trust: How Deregulation has Jeopardized Airline Safety and What You Can do About It*. New York: William Morrow, 1986.

National Transportation Safety Board. *Fatigue, Alcohol, Other Drugs and Medical Factors in Fatal-to-the-Driver Heavy Truck Crashes*. NTSB, 1990.

Owens, S. M., A. J. McBay, and C. E. Cook. "The Use of Marijuana, Ethanol and Other Drugs Among Drivers Killed in Single Vehicle

Crashes." *Journal of Forensic Sciences* 28, no. 2 (1983): 372–79. Reprinted in Rothe, J. P. *The Trucker's World: Risk, Safety and Mobility*. New Brunswick: Transaction Publishers, 1991.

Rigdon, J. E. "Workers Getting Sick and Tired of Overtime." *Toronto Globe and Mail*, Oct. 1994, p. B4. Reprinted from *Wall Street Journal*.

Rothe, J. P. *The Trucker's World: Risk, Safety and Mobility*. New Brunswick: Transaction Publishers, 1991.

Stampi, C. "Ultrashort Sleep/Wake Patterns and Sustained Performance." In Dinges, D. F. and R. J. Broughton, eds. *Sleep and Alertness: Chronobiological, Behavioral and Medical Aspects of Napping*. New York: Raven, 1989.

Stampi, C., et al. "Ultrashort Sleep Strategies During Sustained Operations." In Costa, G. et al., eds. *Shiftwork: Health, Sleep and Performance*. Proceedings of the Ninth International Symposium on Night and Shift Work, 1989.

Terhune, K. and J. Fell. "The Role of Alcohol, Marijuana and Other Drugs in the Accidents of Injured Drivers." National Highway Traffic Safety Administration Report no. HS-806-181. Washington, D.C.: U.S. Department of Transportation, 1982. Reprinted in Rothe, J. P. *The Trucker's World: Risk, Safety and Mobility*. New Brunswick: Transaction Publishers, 1991.

Tobler, I. "Napping and Polyphasic Sleep in Mammals." In Dinges, D. F. and R. J. Broughton, eds. *Sleep and Alertness: Chronobiological, Behavioral and Medical Aspects of Napping*. New York: Raven, 1989.

U.S. House. Committee Investigating US Steel Corp. *Hearings*. 62nd Congress, 1912.

Warren et. al "Characteristics of Fatally Injured Drivers Testing Positive For Drugs Other Than Alcohol." In Proceedings of Eighth International Conference on Alcohol, Drugs and Traffic Safety,

Stockholm, Sweden, June 1988. Reprinted in Rothe, J. P. *The Trucker's World: Risk, Safety and Mobility.* New Brunswick: Transaction Publishers, 1991.

We invite you to read other self-help books from Whole Person Associates. They are available from booksellers or direct from the publisher. Call 800-247-6789 for a complete catalog.

**Kicking Your Stress Habits:
A Do-it-yourself Guide for Coping with Stress**

by Donald A Tubesing

**Seeking Your Healthy Balance:
A Do-it-yourself Guide to Whole Person Well-being**

by Donald A Tubesing and Nancy Loving Tubesing

**Overcoming Panic, Anxiety, & Phobias:
New Strategies to Free Yourself from Worry and Fear**

by Shirley Babior and Carol Goldman